Investing in Maternal Health

Learning from Malaysia and Sri Lanka

D1004572

Human Development Network

Health, Nutrition, and Population Series

Investing in Maternal Health

Learning from Malaysia and Sri Lanka

Indra Pathmanathan

Jerker Liljestrand

Jo. M. Martins

Lalini C. Rajapaksa

Craig Lissner

Amala de Silva

Swarna Selvaraju

Prabha Joginder Singh

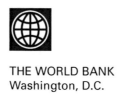

THE WORLD BANK

Washington, D.C.

ISBN 0-8213-5362-4

Library of Congress Cataloging-in-Publication Data *has been applied for.*

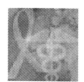

Contents

Foreword   ix

Acknowledgments   xiii

Executive Summary   xvii

Overview   1

Maternal Mortality Can Be Halved in Developing
    Countries Every 7 to 10 Years   2

Maternal Mortality Reduction Is Affordable
    Regardless of Income Level and Growth Rate   4

Maternal Mortality Declines Rapidly with the
    Provision of a Synergistic Package of Health and
    Social Services That Reach the Poor   5

Governments Can Afford to Provide the Critical
    Elements of Maternity Care Free of Charge to
    the Client   10

Different Tactics Are Needed at Different Stages
    of Health Systems Development   12

Official Recognition of Professional Midwifery Is
    a Crucial Step toward Reducing Maternal
    Mortality   16

Raising the Importance of Maternal Death through
    Recording, Reporting, and Subsequent Advocacy
    Will Improve Program Performance   19

Conclusion   20

Note   21

1 **The Ingredients of Success**   23
   The Conceptual Basis   24
   Aims of the Study   32
   Study Approach   32
   The Evidence   36
   Maternal Mortality Transition: A Model for Action   47
   Conclusion   58
   Notes   59

2 **Malaysia**   61
   Background: Malaysia Today   61
   Political Context   62
   Study Approach   64
   Decline in Maternal Mortality   68
   Key Policies and Program Interventions   73
   Summary   102
   Notes   103

3 **Sri Lanka**   105
   Background: Sri Lanka Today   105
   Political and Social Context   105
   Study Approach   108
   Decline in Maternal Mortality Ratio   112
   Trends in Maternal Mortality Ratio and Female
      Death Rates   113
   Development of Maternal and Child Health
      Services   125
   Implementation of Critical Health Policies   140
   Health System Expenditures, Affordability, and
      Sustainability   145
   Conclusion   150
   Notes   151

Appendixes
1 Data Availability and Quality in Malaysia   153
2 Data Availability and Quality in Sri Lanka   159

3   Assessment of Affordability   163
4   Key Informants   165

References   171

Tables

1   Public Expenditures on Health Services and
    Maternal Health Care, Malaysia and Sri Lanka,
    1950s–90s   5
2   Per Capita Gross National Product for Selected
    Countries   26
3   Amount of Time to Halve Maternal Mortality
    Ratio, Malaysia and Sri Lanka, 1949–92   36
4   Key Health Features, Malaysia and Sri Lanka,
    1940–61   44
5   Public Expenditures on Health Services and
    Maternal Health Care, Malaysia and Sri Lanka,
    1950s–90s   56
6   Malaysia at a Glance   62
7   Amount of Time to Halve the Maternal Mortality
    Ratio, Peninsular Malaysia, 1933–97   68
8   Maternal Mortality Ratio, by Ethnic Group,
    Peninsular Malaysia, 1957–90   69
9   Overview of Health Service Capacity and Skilled
    Attendance during Childbirth, Peninsular
    Malaysia, 1949–95   72
10 Total Fertility Rates, by Ethnic Group, Peninsular
    Malaysia, 1957–97   78
11 Expenditures on Public Health, Malaysia,
    1946–95   79
12 Estimated Public Sector Expenditures on
    Maternal Health Care, Malaysia, 1971–95   81
13 Trends in Expenditures for Maternal Health Care,
    Malaysia, 1946–95   87
14 Sri Lanka at a Glance   106
15 Trends in Adult Literacy, Sri Lanka, 1901–91   109
16 Time to Halve the Maternal Mortality Ratio,
    Sri Lanka, 1930–96   112

17 Deliveries with Skilled Attendance and Maternal
    Mortality Ratio, 1939–95   115

18 Deliveries in the Private Sector, Sri Lanka,
    1981–93   117

19 Decline in Cause-Specific Maternal Mortality
    Ratio, Sri Lanka, 1942–52, 1955–70,
    and 1980–96   120

20 Development of Government-Employed Birth
    Attendants, Sri Lanka, 1930–95   120

21 Contraceptive Prevalence Rate, Sri Lanka,
    1975–2000   122

22 Development of Maternal-Health-Care-Related
    Infrastructure, Sri Lanka, 1931–95   128

23 Categories of Institution, Sri Lanka   129

24 Place of Delivery by Monthly Family Income,
    Sri Lanka, 1982   142

25 Place of Delivery by Sector, Sri Lanka, 1982   143

26 Maternal Health Care Expenditures, Sri Lanka,
    1950–99   147

27 Public and Private Health Services, Sri Lanka,
    1953–96   148

Figures

 1 Maternal Mortality Ratio, Sri Lanka, 1930–95   2

 2 Maternal Mortality Ratio, Malaysia, 1950–99   3

 3 Maternal Mortality Ratio and Expenditure
    on Health as a Percentage of Gross Domestic
    Product in Countries That Have Gross National
    Product Comparable Per Capita to Sri Lanka's   6

 4 Maternal Mortality Ratio and Expenditure
    on Health as a Percentage of Gross Domestic
    Product in Countries That Have Gross National
    Product Comparable Per Capita to Malaysia's   7

 5 Maternal Deaths as the Proportion of Deaths
    among Women of Reproductive Age, Sri Lanka
    and Malaysia, 1950–2000   8

 6 Maternal Mortality Ratio in Less-Developed States
    Compared to Other States, Peninsular Malaysia,
    1970–97   9

7 Maternal Mortality Ratio and Skilled Attendance
at Birth, 1995: Countries with Gross National
Product Comparable to That of Malaysia in
the Early 1960s   12

8 Maternal Mortality Ratio and Skilled Attendance
at Birth, 1995: Countries with Gross National
Product Comparable to That of Sri Lanka in
the Early 1960s   13

9 Maternal Mortality Ratio, 1919–20, in Countries
with Deliveries Predominantly Assisted by
Midwives, Doctors, or Both   17

10 Determinants of Health-Sector Outcomes   27

11 Maternal Mortality Ratio, Malaysia and Sri Lanka,
1950–99   37

12 Critical Elements of Maternal Health Care   41

13 Maternal Mortality Ratio and Percentage of Live
Births with Skilled Attendance, Malaysia,
1949–95   45

14 Maternal Mortality Ratio and Percentage of Live
Births with Skilled Attendance, Sri Lanka,
1930–96   46

15 Maternal Mortality Transition: A Model for Action   48

16 Total Fertility Rate and Maternal Mortality Ratio,
Malaysia, 1957–95   52

17 Total Fertility Rate and Maternal Mortality Ratio,
Sri Lanka, 1952–95   53

18 Neonatal Mortality Rates, Malaysia and Sri Lanka,
1938–99   54

19 Place of Birth and Birth Attendance, Peninsular
Malaysia, 1949–95   71

20 Phases of Health Systems Development for
Maternal Health as Related to Reduction in
Maternal Mortality Ratio, 1933–97   74

21 Admissions to Public Sector Hospitals for
Complications of Pregnancy, Peninsular
Malaysia, 1971–95   95

22 Public Operating Expenditures on Maternal
Health Services as Percentage of Gross
Domestic Product, Malaysia, 1971–95   100

23 Public Capital Expenditures on Maternal Health
    Services as Percentage of Gross Domestic
    Product, Malaysia, 1971–95   101

24 Maternal Mortality Rates and Female Death Rates,
    Ages 15–49, Sri Lanka, 1950–96   114

25 Deliveries in Specialized Units, Medical Offices,
    and Primary-Level Government Institutions,
    Sri Lanka, 1984–99   116

26 Maternal Mortality Ratio Attributed to
    Hypertensive Disease and Sepsis, 1930–96   119

27 Maternal Mortality Ratio Attributed to
    Hemorrhage, Sri Lanka, 1930–95   121

28 Maternal Mortality Ratio and Total Fertility Rate,
    Sri Lanka, 1930–95   123

29 Age-specific Fertility Rates, Sri Lanka, 1962–2000   124

30 Age-specific Maternal Mortality Ratio, Sri Lanka,
    1954–96   125

31 Expenditure on Maternal Health Services as
    Percentage of Gross Domestic Product,
    Sri Lanka, 1950–99   146

Boxes

1 Midwives and Nurse–Midwives in the 1960s and
   1970s   90

2 Midwifery Practice in Small Hospitals in the 1960s
   and 1970s   92

3 The Referral Chain   96

4 We Are Proud of Our Public Health Midwives   134

Foreword

Of the 515,000 maternal deaths that occur every year, 99 percent take place in developing countries. Women in the developing world have a 1 in 48 chance of dying from pregnancy-related causes; the ratio in developed countries is 1 in 1,800. For every woman who dies, another 30–50 women suffer injury, infection, or disease. In developing countries, pregnancy-related complications are among the leading causes of death and disability for women, ages 15–49. Of all the human development indicators, the greatest discrepancy between developed and developing countries is in maternal health.

Key interventions to improve maternal health and reduce maternal mortality are known. They include complementary, mutually reinforcing strategies: mobilizing political commitment and an enabling policy environment; investing in social and economic development such as female education, poverty reduction, and improving women's status; offering family planning services; providing quality antenatal care, skilled attendance during childbirth, and availability of emergency obstetric services for pregnancy complications; and strengthening the health system and community involvement. The challenge has been to implement these interventions in environments where political commitment, policies, and institutions and health systems have been weak. Although some countries—including very poor ones—have been successful in reducing maternal mortality, progress in many countries remains slow.

As a way to assist countries in their efforts to improve maternal health and reduce maternal mortality, we are publishing two volumes, *Investing in Maternal Health: Learning from Malaysia and Sri Lanka,* and *Reducing Maternal Mortality: Learning from Bolivia, China, Egypt, Honduras, Indonesia, Jamaica, and Zimbabwe,* on success stories and lessons learned in improving health and reducing maternal mortality in a range of developing countries. The first book is based on the experiences of Malaysia and Sri Lanka during the past five to six decades. The second book discusses the more recent lessons from Bolivia, China (Yunnan), Egypt, Honduras, Indonesia, Jamaica, and Zimbabwe. These countries have made important strides in improving maternal health, and these books outline what worked and what did not.

The studies of maternal health in Malaysia and Sri Lanka started at a time when maternal mortality was still very high in these two countries. It presents the strategies used over the past half century to reverse this trend, including a supportive policy environment and commitment; professionalizing midwifery and ensuring skilled attendance during childbirth; strengthening health systems; introducing civil registration; and improving quality and access to care through rural midwives with closely linked back-up emergency obstetric services. Issues such as the appropriate mix of private versus public expenditures and enabling intersectoral policies are also discussed.

The case studies of Bolivia, China, Egypt, Honduras, Indonesia, Jamaica, and Zimbabwe address the issue of how maternal mortality can be reduced significantly over the course of a single decade, and which key strategies were used in these countries to achieve this reduction. These case studies also inform the current debate on whether it is wiser to invest first in skilled birth attendants, or in the care of obstetric emergencies, or both at once. The analysis also shows how strong safe motherhood policies can have an impact.

For its part, the World Bank has been strongly committed to improving maternal health and reducing maternal mortality for more than a decade and a half. The World Bank was a founding member of the Safe Motherhood Initiative in 1987 and has backed the Program of Action of the 1994 International Conference on Population and

Development (ICPD). More recently, the Bank has embraced the Millennium Development Goals that were agreed to in September 2000, and they have made maternal health one of its top corporate priorities.

Accordingly, we hope that the experiences described in these two volumes will provide a timely contribution of hard evidence regarding what works as we scale-up efforts to achieve the Millennium Development Goal of improving maternal health. In this sense, it is our aim that these materials help to raise the quality and effectiveness of national programs for safe motherhood backed by developing country governments and the donor community. We will endeavor, too, to ensure that the World Bank simultaneously expands its own support of this important cause.

Robert M. Hecht
Acting Sector Director
Health, Nutrition, and Population

Acknowledgments

This study is the product of intensive teamwork. The authors are deeply indebted to local and international experts who have provided guidance and shared their experience and expertise.

Tan Sri Dato Dr. Abu Bakar Suleiman, former director general of health, Malaysia, and Dr. N. W. Vidyasagara, former director, Family Health, Sri Lanka, were senior advisers to the studies in Malaysia and Sri Lanka, respectively. The studies would not have been possible without their personal support and encouragement.

The governments of Malaysia and Sri Lanka provided strong support for the study. The director of Family Health Services of the Ministry of Health, Malaysia, and the director general of Health Services in Sri Lanka facilitated the study through their interest, administrative support, and access to critical data sources.

Several experts who have held key positions in the governments of Malaysia and Sri Lanka provided input to conceptualize the study and identify data sources; they also shared their personal experience and perceptions as key informants. Several of these health professionals were active in the field beginning in the 1950s and later served as health care managers at various levels of the health care system. Their detailed accounts corroborated and expanded on information from other sources.

The key informants for Malaysia were Abdul Khalid Sahan, Abu Bakar Suleiman, Raja Ahmad Nordin, Ajima Hassan, Ali Hamzah, Rebecca John, K. Kananatu, S. Maheswaran, Alex Matthews, M. S.

Murthy, Thomas Ng Khoon Fong, Raj Karim, Ravindran Jegasothy, and A. Tharmaratnam.

In Sri Lanka, the key informants were A. M. L. Beligaswatte, N.C. de Costa, Dulcie de Silva and team from the National Institute of Health Sciences, Nandrani de Zoysa, Joe Fernando, G. Gamalath, Godfrey Gunathilleke, Anoma Jayathilake, Siva Obeysekara, Lakshman Senanayake, N. W. Vidyasagara, Kusum Wickramasuriya, Hiranthi Wijemanne, and Sybil Wijesinghe.

Much time, patience, and persistent effort is required for hunting down data from reports archived since the 1940s, coming to grips with what the data stand for, and reviewing definitions used at different time periods. In Malaysia, key officials in the Ministry of Health and the Economic Planning Unit of the Prime Minister's Department provided valuable information and access to key documents. The following people assisted the authors with data management for the study: Atiya Abdul Sallam, Low Wah Yun, Ng Man San, Noorliza Noordin, Vanaja Palanisamy, and Wong Yut Lin. In Sri Lanka, the director general of Health Services, the librarian of the Department of Census and Statistics, and the medical statistician and staff provided valuable information and access to documents; Padmal de Silva, Chaminda Egodage, Risintha Premaratne, and Asoka Weerasinghe performed much of the data collection and management.

Lennarth Nystrom of Umea University, Sweden, reviewed the data and provided invaluable guidance on data analysis and presentation.

Within the World Bank, Sadia Chowdhury and Joanne Epp have provided invaluable support at different stages of the study.

We are indebted to the peer reviewers, who took the time to read and provide us with comments and suggestions: Staffan Bergstrom (Karolinska Institute, Stockholm); David Dunlop (Dartmouth University); Petra ten Hoope-Bender (International Confederation of Midwives); Marge Koblinsky (North American Consortium for IMMPACT, Johns Hopkins Bloomberg School of Public Health); Charlotte Leighton (Abt Associates); Matthews Mathai (Christian Medical College, Vellore); Della Sherratt (WHO); Anne Tinker (Save the Children); and Isabel Danel, Elizabeth Lule, Anthony

Measham, Thomas W. Merrick, and Khama Rogo (all at the World Bank).

The funding for this study was generously provided by the Swedish International Development Authority and the Government of the Netherlands.

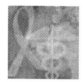

Executive Summary

This study provides the most comprehensive and detailed analysis available on the factors behind the decline in maternal mortality in Malaysia and Sri Lanka in the past 50 to 60 years and the magnitude of health system expenditures on maternal health. The study synthesizes findings from various previous reports with new data collected from archives and from interviews with key informants. The combined data provide the basis for the analysis and conclusions.

The main findings are that a modest investment in maternal health services, combined with other poverty reduction measures, leads to a fairly rapid decline in the maternal mortality ratio (MMR), defined as the number of maternal deaths per 100,000 live births. The strategies of Malaysia and Sri Lanka changed over time, from an initial emphasis on expanding the provision of services, especially in underserved areas, to increasing utilization and, finally, to emphasizing the improvement of quality. Removing financial barriers to maternal care for clients was an important step in both countries. Care of obstetric emergencies at the referral (hospital) level was developed in conjunction with, and closely interwoven with, the gradually increased access to skilled birth attendance, a concept that refers to deliveries by clinically trained midwives, nurse–midwives, or doctors. Professional midwives constitute the backbone of maternal care in Malaysia and Sri Lanka. Recording and reporting of maternal deaths was a prerequisite to addressing maternal mortality reduction in both countries.

The seven main conclusions are summarized in the overview.

In summary, MMR reduction in developing countries is feasible with modest public expenditures when appropriate policies are adopted, focused wisely, and adapted incrementally in response to environmental conditions and systems capacities.

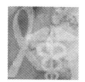

Overview

In recent decades, global maternal mortality has not declined significantly, even though the world has seen huge improvements in health, survival, and fertility. Fifteen years of Safe Motherhood initiatives have provided better recognition of the impact of maternal deaths and the vulnerability of the poor. Good evidence is available on which clinical interventions work and which do not, but less is known about how best to implement strategies to reduce national and local levels of maternal mortality under conditions that prevail in developing countries. The difference in maternal mortality between the industrialized and the developing world is greater than any other development indicator. The apparent lack of progress has generated a sense of despondency. Is it possible to reduce maternal mortality in developing countries? Can progress be achieved within time periods sufficiently short to sustain the commitment of policymakers? Can maternal health keep pace with improvements in other human development indicators?

Malaysia and Sri Lanka are among the developing countries that have successfully reduced maternal mortality during the past few decades to levels comparable with those of many industrialized countries. Recognizing that Sri Lanka had the advantage of early gains in female literacy and Malaysia had the advantage of beginning with a relatively stronger economy, can their implementation experience benefit other developing countries? Analysis of their experience provides evidence to support several key messages of interest to policymakers and international development agencies.

Maternal Mortality Can Be Halved in Developing Countries Every 7 to 10 Years

Rapid declines in maternal mortality took place in Malaysia and Sri Lanka even before the 1950s, when both countries had relatively low gross national product (GNP) per capita. At that time Malaysia's female literacy was low (17 percent), and the male–female literacy ratio was 0.32. Under those conditions, both countries halved their maternal mortality ratio (MMR), defined as the number of maternal deaths per 100,000 live births, with impressive speed, as shown in figures 1 and 2.

An initial period of rapid decline took place; MMR was reduced by half within 3 years in Sri Lanka (1947–50) and within 7 years in Malaysia (1950–57). Subsequent to the initial rapid decline, it took each country 13 years to slice MMR in half again. During this period access to basic health care, including critical elements of maternal

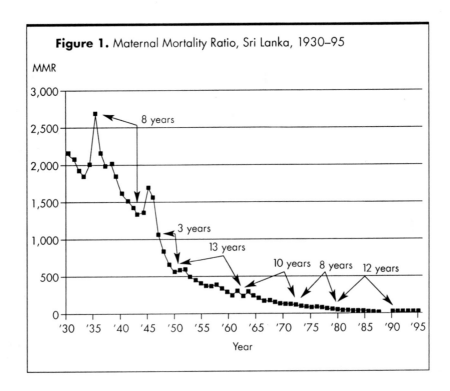

Figure 1. Maternal Mortality Ratio, Sri Lanka, 1930–95

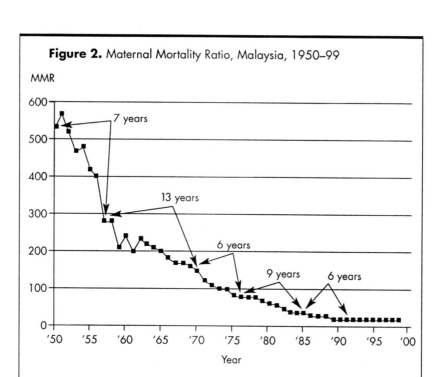

Figure 2. Maternal Mortality Ratio, Malaysia, 1950–99

health care, was improved for the bulk of the rural population through a widespread rural health network. In subsequent decades both Malaysia and Sri Lanka systematically applied stepwise strategies to improve organizational and clinical management and reduced their MMR by 50 percent every 6–12 years.

These achievements mirror the experience of several industrialized countries and some developing countries. For example, MMR in Sweden declined from 600 to 230 per 100,000 live births from 1870–95, when specific efforts made professional birthing care widely available. In Thailand, MMR decreased from 430 to 100 between 1960 and 1980. Both Sweden and Thailand had large poor populations during these periods along with widespread illiteracy and significant burdens of infectious disease and malnutrition. Despite these burdens, the countries rapidly reduced MMR from high levels through focused and sustained efforts (De Brouwere and Van Lerberghe 2001).

Maternal Mortality Reduction Is Affordable Regardless of Income Level and Growth Rate

Sri Lanka is a low-income country, whereas Malaysia has been among the middle-income countries. In the late 1950s, Sri Lanka's GNP per capita was US$270 (1995 US$ equivalent) and Malaysia's was US$965; in both countries, about half of the households were below the poverty line. It is apparent that both countries were much poorer when they commenced their efforts to reduce maternal mortality. The two countries had considerably different income levels and have experienced different rates of economic growth.

Maternal health care in both countries has been provided largely by the public sector. Throughout the period when MMR decline was rapid and sustained, analysis of public finances shows that total public expenditures on health care were modest: since the 1950s, they have amounted to only about 1.4 to 1.8 percent of gross domestic product (GDP) in Malaysia and an average of 1.8 percent of GDP in Sri Lanka. In Malaysia, expenditures on maternal health care in public hospitals and maternal and child health (MCH) services in the community were a humble 0.38 percent of GDP, on average, while in Sri Lanka expenditures were even lower, at 0.23 percent of GDP (table 1). Note that Sri Lanka had completed an initial investment in building for its extensive health infrastructure of clinics and hospitals in rural areas prior to the 1950s; Malaysia's rural health service was strengthened and hospitals were upgraded and expanded after Independence was achieved in 1957.

A comparison of Sri Lanka's and Malaysia's MMR to that of countries with similar per capita GNP (based on "purchasing power pari-

Low- and middle-income countries with substantially different levels of income and growth rates can reduce maternal mortality.

Table 1. Public Expenditures on Health Services and Maternal Health Care, Malaysia and Sri Lanka, 1950s–90s

PERIOD	MALAYSIA PUBLIC EXPENDITURES (%GDP)		SRI LANKA PUBLIC EXPENDITURES (%GDP)	
	TOTAL HEALTH SERVICES	MATERNAL HEALTH CARE[a]	TOTAL HEALTH SERVICES	MATERNAL HEALTH CARE[a]
1950–55	—	—	1.71	0.28
1956–60	1.54	—	2.29	0.28
1961–65	1.71	—	2.11	0.31
1966–70	—	—	2.10	0.29
1971–75	1.79	0.32	1.81	0.28
1976–80	1.63	0.36	1.62	0.23
1981–85	1.59	0.41	1.30	0.16
1986–90	1.51	0.40	1.72	0.19
1991–95	1.44	0.37	1.52	0.17
1996–99	—	—	1.56	0.14
1950–99	—	—	1.79	0.23

— Not available.

Note: Data may not sum to totals because of rounding.

[a] Includes hospital care for deliveries, complications of pregnancy, and community-based maternal and child health services.

ty of national currencies") indicates that Sri Lanka (figure 3) has obtained better results than its peers (figure 8) for a lower health expenditure per capita (figure 3), and Malaysia (figure 4) has attained the same or better maternal mortality outcomes at a much lower level of health expenditures per capita. This finding is consistent with other evidence: it is not the level of expenditure, but the specific interventions, that make the difference in lowering maternal mortality.

Maternal Mortality Declines Rapidly with the Provision of a Synergistic Package of Health and Social Services That Reach the Poor

The governments of Malaysia and Sri Lanka consistently implemented human development programs that reached underprivileged groups, such as the rural poor (both countries), disadvantaged ethnic groups and less developed states (Malaysia), and plantation workers

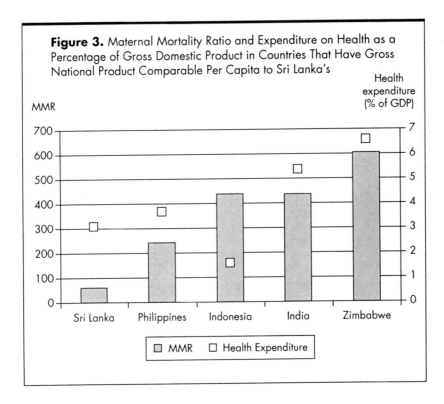

Figure 3. Maternal Mortality Ratio and Expenditure on Health as a Percentage of Gross Domestic Product in Countries That Have Gross National Product Comparable Per Capita to Sri Lanka's

(Sri Lanka). The development programs were based on the concept that basic health care acts in synergy with basic education, water, and sanitation and integrated rural development. Women's involvement was emphasized, both implicitly and, sometimes, explicitly, and gender equity was a priority in both countries. Maternal health elements were implemented in a basic health care package that included malaria control, child health, and family planning.

Thus, in Malaysia, within the first 18 years after Independence, female life expectancy increased from 58 to 69 years and maternal mortality declined by 70 percent. Integrated rural development provided improved access to basic education, rural roads, sanitation, and water supply. Key health messages, including those concerning the use of skilled attendance[1] during childbirth, were provided through rural development initiatives such as adult education classes. Fur-

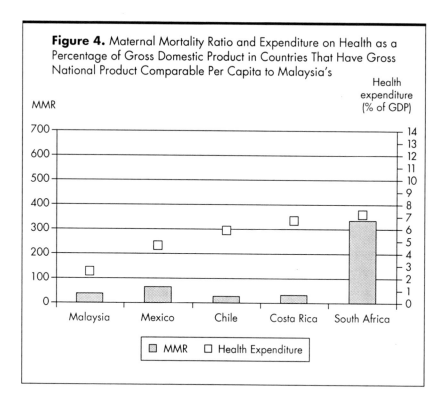

Figure 4. Maternal Mortality Ratio and Expenditure on Health as a Percentage of Gross Domestic Product in Countries That Have Gross National Product Comparable Per Capita to Malaysia's

thermore, rural roads improved access to rural health facilities and facilitated transportation of obstetric emergencies.

Similar advances occurred in Sri Lanka. For example, female literacy increased from 44 percent in 1946 to 71 percent in 1971, and the male–female literacy ratio narrowed. Small cottage hospitals and maternity homes staffed with public health midwives were opened rapidly and were widely distributed in rural areas. Family planning services were integrated into the MCH program. Ambulance services were rapidly expanded.

The trend in maternal deaths as a proportion of the deaths of women of reproductive age is a measure of the success attributable to interventions specifically related to maternal health. The success of maternal health care interventions in Malaysia and Sri Lanka is evident from the large fall in the number of maternal deaths as a

- Maternal health care is particularly effective when provided within a synergistic package of services.
- The package needs to reach the poor.
- Fertility reduction is associated with MMR decline at certain stages of health systems development.

proportion of the total number of women's deaths in reproductive ages. In Malaysia this proportion declined from about 10 percent to 1 percent from the 1950s to the 1990s, and the fall was even larger in Sri Lanka, as shown in figure 5.

Furthermore, evidence from Malaysia indicates that when an appropriate package of services is directed to the rural and poor, poorer groups rapidly achieve low maternal mortality levels that are

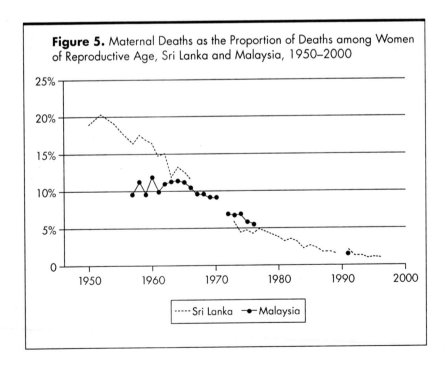

Figure 5. Maternal Deaths as the Proportion of Deaths among Women of Reproductive Age, Sri Lanka and Malaysia, 1950–2000

equivalent to mortality levels among their better-off counterparts. Malaysian states that had high household poverty levels initially had higher MMR than did states with lower poverty. Figure 6 demonstrates how the difference in MMR levels between states was rapidly narrowed and eliminated.

As in Malaysia, wide variations in maternal mortality rates existed between districts in Sri Lanka during the period 1962–71. By 1980, however, the MMR in all districts converged, and the variation from district to district was minimal. This leveling indicates relative improvement of the health services in less developed areas of the country (Rodrigo 1987). Within a 10-year period of focused efforts in Sri Lanka, the proportion of women in Sri Lankan tea estates who previously did not have skilled attendance during childbirth declined from 40 to 10 percent (Vidyasagara 1983).

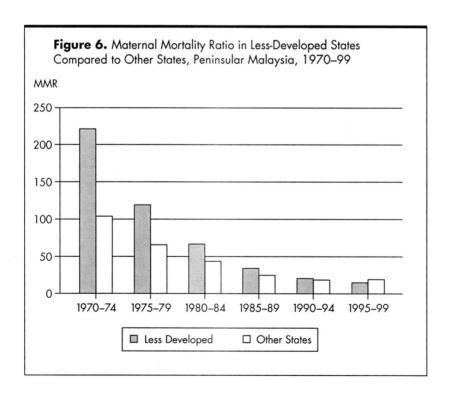

Figure 6. Maternal Mortality Ratio in Less-Developed States Compared to Other States, Peninsular Malaysia, 1970–99

Fertility decline, as evidenced by the total fertility rate (TFR)—the average number of children that a woman age 15 can expect to bear if she lives until at least age 50—only began after 1960 in both countries. Thus, the initial steep reduction in MMR, which took place in the period from 1945–60, was not significantly associated with fertility decline. Since 1960, however, TFR has fallen gradually in both countries in a linear relationship with the MMR decline. Both the reduction of pregnancies in older women who had borne many children and the reduction of very early teen pregnancies may have contributed to MMR reduction in this period. Decreased reliance on unsafe abortion, due partly to improved contraceptive access, probably also contributed.

Governments Can Afford to Provide the Critical Elements of Maternity Care Free of Charge to the Client

Both Malaysia and Sri Lanka provided maternity care free to clients who could not pay for services. Evidence from Malaysia indicates that neither formal nor informal user fees were factors that significantly influenced utilization of hospital services (Young and others 1980). In both countries, household income levels have not hindered access to health care. (Hammer and others 1995; Vidyasagara 1983).

Although formal user fees for certain health services appear to be acceptable for many users in various settings, exceptions exist. For example, in some countries care for sudden, life-threatening conditions, such as serious complications during childbirth, is often denied to poor families. Fee-exemption schemes generally do not function well under such circumstances. Furthermore, informal fees for acute maternal conditions can be high, even ruinous to the family, and can be effective deterrents to the seeking of care (Nahar and Costello 1998). Where transportation schemes for obstetric emergencies have not been organized, physical access is often limited due to cost and access to transportation.

It is interesting to review the use of skilled attendance in selected countries that had economic situations similar to Malaysia and Sri Lanka 40 to 45 years ago. Although on average, at least 40 percent of

- Removing financial barriers to care is a key element in success.
- Appropriate policies and programs make maternal health care affordable to countries and clients.

women in the selected countries use skilled attendance today, large disparities exist between the wealthiest and poorest groups. Although Malaysia and Sri Lanka do not have data on the use of skilled attendance in different wealth quintiles, other evidence demonstrates that in these two countries, the poor have the same access to skilled attendance as their wealthier counterparts. This finding suggests that removal of financial barriers to access to maternal health care would accelerate reduction of MMR.

Apart from initial capital investment in building facilities that are accessible to rural communities, the major expenditure in maternal health care is the operational cost associated with the human resources needed to provide services. Malaysia and Sri Lanka were able to afford widespread access to maternal health care by using a judicious mix of health personnel. The bulk of maternal health care is provided by well-trained but relatively low-cost midwives, who are adequately supplied and equipped and are closely supervised and supported by nurse–midwives and much smaller numbers of medical doctors (see chapters 2 and 3).

Furthermore, in both countries, the levels of capital expenditure that reflect market prices of construction and equipment remained relatively stable during the period under review. However, operating expenses that mirror the number and salary rates of public servants show a declining trend in the case of Sri Lanka and a later, smaller decline in Malaysia. This decrease was achieved despite the increasing numbers of health professionals employed. The lowering of salary rates of health professionals in relation to GDP per capita allowed the engagement of more public servants without a proportional increase in operating expenditures.

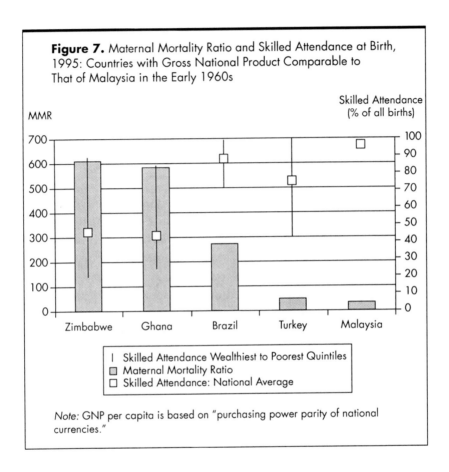

Figure 7. Maternal Mortality Ratio and Skilled Attendance at Birth, 1995: Countries with Gross National Product Comparable to That of Malaysia in the Early 1960s

Legend:
| Skilled Attendance Wealthiest to Poorest Quintiles
▨ Maternal Mortality Ratio
□ Skilled Attendance: National Average

Note: GNP per capita is based on "purchasing power parity of national currencies."

Different Tactics Are Needed at Different Stages of Health Systems Development

Today, developing countries are at different phases of health systems development. Historically, when Malaysia and Sri Lanka evolved through phases that were roughly equivalent to the situation prevalent in developing countries today, various tactics were used to implement the critical elements of maternal health care. The tactics were implemented in a stepwise fashion in accordance with the needs and conditions of the evolving health systems. The critical ele-

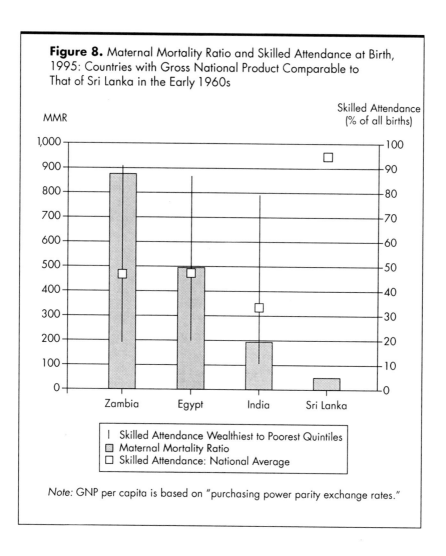

Figure 8. Maternal Mortality Ratio and Skilled Attendance at Birth, 1995: Countries with Gross National Product Comparable to That of Sri Lanka in the Early 1960s

Legend:
| Skilled Attendance Wealthiest to Poorest Quintiles
▨ Maternal Mortality Ratio
☐ Skilled Attendance: National Average

Note: GNP per capita is based on "purchasing power parity exchange rates."

ments in the successive phases can be characterized as (a) establishing solid foundations for effective maternity care, (b) increasing access to such care, and (c) subsequently ensuring appropriate utilization of available services through improved quality.

The *foundation* that supported development of effective maternal health care included professionalization of midwifery, civil registra-

Transition from high to low MMR passes through evolutionary phases characterized by:

- High MMR with low levels of skilled attendance
- Declining MMR with medium levels of skilled attendance
- High levels of skilled attendance with acceptable MMR or high levels of skilled attendance with plateau or unacceptable levels of MMR.

Strategies to reduce MMR during different phases would need to evolve as follows:

- Establishing foundations for effective maternal health services: professionalized midwifery, monitoring systems, and advocacy
- Improving access for rural and disadvantaged communities and community mobilization
- Improving utilization of available services through improved quality and client empowerment.

tion of births, and use of compiled reports of maternal deaths to draw attention to the seriousness of the problem and replicate elements of local success.

When the health systems were relatively underdeveloped, the key focus of implementation was on *improving access* to treatment of maternal complications. Financial, geographic, and cultural barriers to access were addressed in Malaysia and Sri Lanka by making competent professional midwives and supervisory nurse–midwives widely available in rural areas, ensuring them a steady supply of appropriate drugs and equipment, linking them to back-up services, and improving communication and transportation. These respected midwives helped overcome cultural barriers through links with the communities and partnerships with traditional birth attendants. They assisted deliveries in homes and small rural hospitals and gave initial treatment to women who had complications. Evidence suggests that their impact spread well beyond the women they actually attended. Because the midwives were locally available and well respected, they received and responded to calls for help from the community, even from women who developed complications while being attended by unskilled persons, and they made sure that women with serious complications reached appropriate facilities for further care.

Simultaneously, the facilities were strengthened to care for complications; some rural facilities provided basic essential obstetric care, and others had surgical facilities that offered full comprehensive essential obstetric care. At that time, the number of doctors was relatively small. For example, Malaysia had only one doctor per 15,500 births. A few committed doctors in small hospitals provided backup for a substantial number of midwives. Within a decade, it was possible to increase skilled birth attendance to greater than 40 percent and to halve maternal mortality. The impact of these measures is evidenced by the 65 percent decline in deaths from sepsis and 77 percent decline in deaths from hypertensive disease in Sri Lanka.

As access increased, the countries further strengthened supportive supervision and accountability through training, better organizational management, and mobilization of communities. Midwife-assisted home births initially increased, then declined. Simultaneously, institutionalization of births increased in hospitals, clinics, and nursing homes that provided either basic or referral-level obstetric care (see figures 13 and 14 in chapter 1).

Once a wide network of accessible services was established, the focus shifted to *improved utilization* of available services through quality improvement processes and to empowering clients to expect quality services and use them appropriately. Measures encompassed strengthening clinical and organizational management, including implementation of increasingly sophisticated monitoring systems. Referral mechanisms became effective, and the demand increased for childbirth in more sophisticated hospitals in the public and private sectors. Progressively more sophisticated and formal quality improvement mechanisms were introduced with strong support from management and clinical leaders and are being expanded to include the private sector.

During all phases, antenatal care and home visits have been the major channel for promoting the use of skilled attendance during childbirth. Postpartum care and postabortion care have developed concurrently with the expansion of the delivery of care. The emphasis on professional attention during the postpartum week—through home visits and defined procedures for managing postpartum complications—has been important. The need for postabortion care has diminished as the problem of unsafe abortion has been reduced.

Official Recognition of Professional Midwifery Is a Crucial Step toward Reducing Maternal Mortality

Evidence from Malaysia and Sri Lanka indicates that the competence, status, and role of midwives and nurse–midwives have been central features in MMR reduction. An outstanding feature of both countries is the long-standing professional status of midwifery. Since the 1930s, Malaysia and Sri Lanka have defined the "skilled attendant" as a clinically trained, certified, and legally registered midwife; a nurse–midwife; or a medical doctor. Thus, in the late 1940s and 1950s, when investments in maternal health care were given priority in the newly independent countries, the required competencies for the professional midwife had been defined and accepted, and there was experience in how to train this cadre of health workers. Both countries established early the need for close and competent supervision and, accordingly, trained and placed professional nurse–midwives. The special identity and competence of these workers are well recognized by communities and professionals in both countries.

The midwife and supervisory nurse–midwife combined credibility, outreach, and connection. The early and massive efforts in competency-based training and placement of midwives in rural areas provided a means of reaching out to rural communities and resulted in the midwives being the frontline primary health care worker. The midwife constituted the first point of contact with the formal health

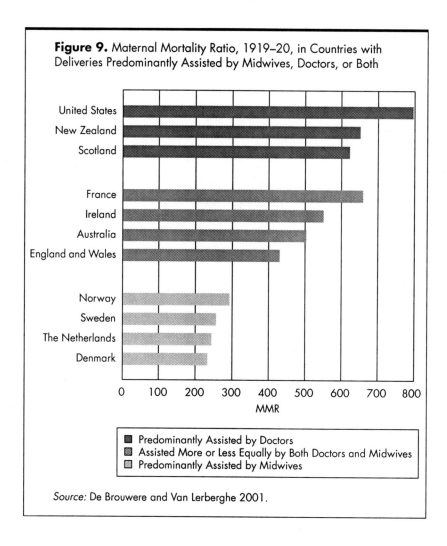

Figure 9. Maternal Mortality Ratio, 1919–20, in Countries with Deliveries Predominantly Assisted by Midwives, Doctors, or Both

Source: De Brouwere and Van Lerberghe 2001.

care system, both through the care that she provided and through her propelling of people further into the health system. Her clinical skills gave her credibility with communities. Thus, communities sought her help to save the lives of women, even if she had not been the actual birth attendant. MMR declined rapidly when the proportion of childbirth with skilled attendance reached about 50 percent.

In a recent review, De Brouwere and Van Lerberghe (2001) explored the issue of professionalization of care delivery and the

Information is an essential foundation for maternal health improvement. It requires:

- Improved civil registration of births and deaths
- Mobilizing communities to provide information on births and deaths
- Improved medical records
- Official investigations of maternal deaths and development of confidential inquiries into maternal deaths
- Production of analytical reports on maternal deaths.

Use of information is critical for success:

- Local information fuels advocacy to mobilize and sustain political commitment and community support
- Subnational monitoring improves program performance.

optimal mixture of professionals. In summary, various experiences show that with the right training, supervision, regulation, and accountability for results, midwives perform well, constitute an effective intervention in reducing MMR (figure 9), and are needed to balance the often poor performance of doctors and hospitals.

Several developing countries have large cadres of workers called midwives, but those workers do not have the necessary clinical competence. Their role is sometimes reduced to counseling and supplying contraceptives and micronutrients, and they may have little clinical credibility. Communities are hardly likely to approach them when life-threatening crises occur. Medical doctors are too distant from rural villages or too expensive for the poor, and some doctors might not possess the necessary obstetric skills. The experiences of Malaysia and Sri Lanka demonstrate how it is possible to train, deploy, and sustain large cadres of clinically competent midwives within relatively short time periods.

Raising the Importance of Maternal Death through Recording, Reporting, and Subsequent Advocacy Will Improve Program Performance

Early in their development, Malaysia and Sri Lanka established civil registration systems for births and deaths independent of the health sector. Various incentives were linked to the reporting in those systems (for example, citizenship, voting, employment, and security). Politicians and leaders were continually confronted with area-specific mortality data, including data on maternal deaths; this information proved to be a powerful lever for initiating and sustaining maternal health programs and other interventions to benefit the poor. This experience is similar to that of many industrialized countries, as discussed by De Brouwere, Tonglet, and Van Lerberghe (1998). For example, the registration of births and deaths in Sweden, begun in 1749, was critically important for interventions to reduce maternal and infant mortality in the 19th century (Hogberg and Wall 1986).

Although registration of deaths and births may not be feasible immediately in many developing countries, alternative measures are possible. For example, most countries in Sub-Saharan Africa give community attention to every death, as in the acquisition of permission for burial. This attention offers a potential starting point for documenting and acting on maternal deaths. Verbal autopsies of the death of women of fertile age can also provide relatively good information on which deaths are maternal (Hoj, Stensballe, and Aaby 1999).

Within the health system, both Malaysia and Sri Lanka instituted systems for maternal death review that evolved as the health system developed. Early reviews involved local investigation of maternal deaths with the participation of local midwives, medical authorities in hospitals and health districts, and the family and community. National- and state-level officials visited villages that had a maternal death; this attention helped local staff, as well as communities, recognize the importance of every maternal death. The review was generally "no blame": everyone involved was clear that the purpose was to learn from each death and try to improve the system to prevent similar deaths (Joe Fernando and Raj Karim, informant interviews). Cause-specific death information was increasingly collected and analyzed, and the data provided the basis for program decisions, such as midwives' active management of the third stage of labor (that is, when the placenta comes out) and use of oxytocics, which are drugs that help contract the womb (Rebecca John and Ajima Hassan, informant interviews). As the number of maternal deaths declined, it became possible to institute full-fledged "confidential inquiries into maternal deaths," which involve professionals at various levels in the public and private sectors. Although the public sector has taken the lead, professional bodies have associated themselves closely, and the "enquiries" are modeled on international practice. Such reviews have become quality improvement tools and have served to improve collaboration between public and private providers (Abu Bakar, Mathews, Jegasothy, and others 1999).

Conclusion

Maternal mortality poses a major challenge in the fight against poverty and premature death, as it impoverishes families and affects child support and development. The Malaysian and Sri Lankan experiences provide evidence that developing countries can reduce maternal mortality successfully. Their efforts show that maternal mortality can be halved every 7–10 years when a synergistic package of health and social services reaches the poor. This is affordable to countries regardless of their income levels or economic growth, and governments can afford to provide the critical elements of maternity care free of charge to their citizens. To a great extent, it is not how much is spent but on what and who gets it that matters most. Raising the importance of maternal deaths through purposeful recording, reporting, analysis and continuing advocacy is essential to improve program performance. The official recognition of professional midwifery is a critical element in reducing maternal mortality. A pragmatic but systematic developmental approach is needed that would address any cultural barriers to health care access and deal appropriately with the interests of traditional birth attendants. This development program would include appropriate transport and communication facilities, guarantee professionalism, and ensure that services are adequately resourced and supervised.

Note

1. The term "skilled attendance" refers to deliveries by clinically trained midwives, nurse–midwives, or doctors.

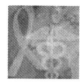

CHAPTER 1

The Ingredients
of Success

The framework for the analysis presented in this chapter is provided by two parallel questions that policymakers in many developing countries face today:

- Are effective maternal health interventions affordable in relatively poor countries?

- How would such interventions be implemented in relatively weak health systems?

Malaysia and Sri Lanka are two of the few developing countries that have relatively good historical data, reports, and a track record of success in reducing maternal mortality. Case studies of the two countries therefore provide sufficient evidence to derive pointers for other developing countries. The experience of Malaysia and Sri Lanka has been presented in conferences and quoted widely in recent years. However, this study presents the first comprehensive, in-depth description and analysis that includes policy analysis, health systems development, trends in utilization of skilled birth attendance and maternal mortality, and public expenditures on maternal health. Recent developments have provided the framework for analysis of the two case studies. First, recognition of the need to focus on poor population segments to speed development has grown internationally, and better understanding exists of how poor countries can support human development. Second, evaluations of the first decade of

Safe Motherhood produced a firmer grasp of which maternal health strategies and interventions work. International agencies are focusing on skilled birth attendance as a critical factor in reducing maternal mortality, and they now have a stronger handle on the dynamics of health policies and programs in improving maternal health.

The Conceptual Basis

National Poverty Reduction Strategy Papers (PRSPs), which demonstrate a commitment to special strategies for improving the circumstances of poor populations, have become a prerequisite for international lending and for conditioning of debt relief for heavily indebted poor countries. The specific interventions in PRSPs strongly emphasize bringing basic services to the poor (World Bank 2000). Core services include basic education and basic health care. The papers emphasize the need to engage women and girls in the development process by ensuring access to basic education and basic health care and directly involving girls and women in the national developmental processes. Poor countries simply cannot afford to ignore the potential capacity of women and their place in national development and poverty reduction. Improving maternal health and reducing the maternal mortality ratio (MMR) is integral to such efforts.

Providing health care services to the poor is an underlying force that has sustained substantial improvements in life expectancy and infant and maternal mortality for both developed and developing countries. Reaching the poor makes sense because low income can be a main factor in low literacy and illness and because better schooling and health may raise productivity and income (Sen 1999).

At least two models have been identified in successful attempts at reducing mortality (Sen 1999). The first is thought to achieve declines in mortality by "growth-mediated" processes that promote employment and increase the use of health care and education, financed by economic growth. The second may be described as a "support-led" process that does not use economic growth but provides appropriate social services, such as health care, education, and other safety-net support. Empirical evidence indicates that under either model, success depends on reaching poor people and enabling them to improve their human and social functioning.

In light of countries' different levels of per capita income and rates of economic growth, the question has often been raised of how poor countries can finance support-led processes that include health care and education. According to economics Nobel laureate Amartya Sen (1999), this is a good question that also

> has a good answer, which lies very considerably in the economics of relative costs. The viability of this support-led process is dependent on the fact that the relevant social services (such as health and basic education) are very *labor intensive*, and thus are relatively inexpensive in poor—and low-wage—economies. A poor economy may *have* less money to spend on health care and education, but it also *needs* less money to spend to provide the same services, which would cost much more in richer countries. (pp. 47–8)

The results of this study illustrate Sen's contention. Both Malaysia and Sri Lanka have been capable of sustaining public expenditures for basic services such as health, in spite of their substantial differences in levels of income per capita and rates of economic growth. Malaysia has about 3 times the amount of Sri Lanka's per capita income and has experienced about 1.5 times the growth rate of Sri Lanka over 35 years (World Bank 2001). Table 2 shows the per capita gross national product (GNP) of these two countries during the late 1950s, when considerable expansion of public expenditures on health care took place, and shows that per capita GNP in 1995 U.S. dollars was comparable to that of many developing countries today.

A major issue in access to skilled attendance[1] is the financial burden that either official or hidden fees may impose on household financial resources, especially in the case of the poor. This question deserves considerable attention because access to maternal health services, as well as transportation, may make the difference during difficult deliveries and complications of pregnancy. If a household is poor, it is unlikely to be able to rely on savings for this purpose, and

Table 2. Per Capita Gross National Product for Selected Countries (1995 US$)

COUNTRY	PER CAPITA GNP
About the time of expansion of public funding for maternal health care	
Sri Lanka (1959)	270
Malaysia (1957)	965
In 1995	
Tanzania	120
Bangladesh	240
Uganda	240
Mali	250
Pakistan	460
Egypt	790
Philippines	1,050

Sources: World Bank 1978, 1981, 1997; Malaysia Department of Statistics 1999; Central Bank of Ceylon 1968–84; Central Bank of Sri Lanka 1986–99.

any credit obtained might be at the cost of future necessities. The barriers posed by formal and informal fees appear to influence the uptake of birthing care more than antenatal care (World Bank 1999). The case studies indicate how this issue was addressed.

Preventing Maternal Deaths

Maternal deaths have devastating and costly effects on children, families, and communities, and they are largely preventable. A complex interaction of various factors contributes to such disastrous outcomes. The dynamic interaction of determinants of health, as outlined in *Poverty-Reduction and the Health-Sector* (Claeson and others 2001), provide the conceptual basis for analyzing the case studies of Malaysia and Sri Lanka (figure 10).

Maternal–newborn health status is the outcome of the dynamic interaction among complex factors. The behavior of households and communities can reduce health complications associated with pregnancy and childbirth. For example, some complications are specific to very young girls who become pregnant and to the effects of the pregnancy on their nutritional status; other complications are associated with the number and frequency of pregnancies. Household and

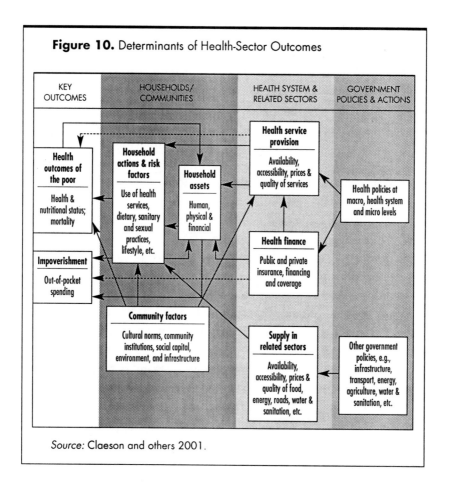

Figure 10. Determinants of Health-Sector Outcomes

| KEY OUTCOMES | HOUSEHOLDS/ COMMUNITIES | HEALTH SYSTEM & RELATED SECTORS | GOVERNMENT POLICIES & ACTIONS |

Health service provision

Health outcomes of the poor

Health & nutritional status; mortality

Household actions & risk factors

Use of health services, dietary, sanitary and sexual practices, lifestyle, etc.

Household assets

Human, physical & financial

Availability, accessibility, prices & quality of services

Health policies at macro, health system and micro levels

Impoverishment

Out-of-pocket spending

Health finance

Public and private insurance, financing and coverage

Community factors

Cultural norms, community institutions, social capital, environment, and infrastructure

Supply in related sectors

Availability, accessibility, prices & quality of food, energy, roads, water & sanitation, etc.

Other government policies, e.g., infrastructure, transport, energy, agriculture, water & sanitation, etc.

Source: Claeson and others 2001.

community decisionmaking and behavior influences these issues, such as whether to seek health care during pregnancy and childbirth, the type of care that is sought, and when care is sought. The status of women in the community influences the dynamics and outcomes of such decisionmaking. The status of women has several dimensions, and no single indicator can measure all of them. However, the difference between male and female literacy rates is one indicator for which data are readily available and is useful for monitoring women's status.

The capacity of a health system to influence maternal health behavior and outcomes depends on its ability to provide timely, effective care and finance it. Health system capacity is influenced by national policies and priorities, which are reflected in resource allocation, monitoring, and regulation. Decisions on investment and utilization of the allocated resources determine the design of the health program, and clinical and organizational management determine the effectiveness of program implementation and interaction with other sectors. For example, national priorities and decisions would determine the types and distribution of health facilities and health personnel, which in turn would influence the proportion of women in the nation who have access to appropriate maternal health services. Effective organizational and clinical management ensures that maternal health services promote healthy pregnancy and childbirth practices, provide a clean and safe environment for childbirth, detect complications, transport women, and manage complications promptly in appropriate facilities.

Other sectors influence health care capacity. The educational sector, water and sanitation, roads and communications, and food security have dynamic interactions with maternal health care and maternal–newborn health. For example, education, particularly girls' education, influences health behavior, including health care seeking. Roads and communications influence geographic access, ease transportation of emergencies during childbirth, and support the capacity of the health care system to improve distribution of skilled health personnel and disseminate information.

These elements provide a framework that has guided the analysis of these two case studies so as to yield conclusions that would be potentially helpful for health professionals and managers, economists, and policymakers.

Causes of Maternal Deaths

Pregnancy and birth are normal life events that usually do not require special clinical intervention. However, about 15 percent of all pregnant women anywhere in the world will experience a potentially life-threatening complication, and 1 to 2 percent of all pregnant women will die as a result of their pregnancy unless they have access to major surgery. About 80 percent of maternal deaths are due to postpartum bleeding, severe infection, obstructed labor (that is, the baby cannot pass through the birth canal due to disproportion or malpresentation), eclampsia, or postabortion complications. Most such deaths are preventable with appropriate medical care. It is evident that having no access to care implies a great risk for pregnant, birthing, and postpartum women and their offspring. This situation explains why women in some Sub-Saharan countries run a lifetime risk of 1 in 8 of a maternal death while women in, for instance, Western Europe have a risk of 1 in 4,800.[2]

Maternal deaths also result from preexisting or coincidental disease aggravated by the pregnancy. The relative importance of indirect causes of death depends on the general health status of the population (for example, the prevalence of malnutrition, malaria, HIV/AIDS, tuberculosis, and heart disease; WHO 1999). Maternal mortality may be prevented to a limited extent by the general improvement of health through factors such as malaria control, improved water and sanitation, adequate nutrition, and better women's education. Addressing such factors in isolation, however, will not reduce MMR to acceptable levels. An often quoted example is that of a religious group in the United States. Pregnant women in this group were generally considered low risk from a demographic and health viewpoint, but their religious beliefs prevented them from receiving medical care. From 1975 to 1982 their MMR was 872 per 100,000 live births, compared with 9 per 100,000 live births in the general population (Kaunitz and others 1984). *Faith Assembly*

Effective Measures: Learning from Developing and Industrialized Countries

The road to MMR reduction in what is labeled the industrialized world has been analyzed and discussed (De Brouwere, Tonglet, and Van Lerberghe 1998). Key components were the professionalization of birthing care, management of emergencies and complications of pregnancy and childbirth, and registration of births and deaths—all backed by a sustained political commitment. The major MMR decline in such countries, however, took place largely before the introduction of modern obstetrics: blood transfusion and antibiotics did not yet exist, and cesarean section was a rarity. Improvements also occurred in countries that had high degrees of literacy, limited malnutrition, and few scourges like malaria. The success stories of developing countries in the past 50 years demand attention and analysis because they are probably most relevant to developing countries today. The case studies of Malaysia and Sri Lanka explore whether the measures that led to success in industrialized countries could be applied or adapted to developing countries.

Skilled Attendance during Childbirth

Professionalization of birthing care is a complex concept, and the term "skilled attendance" has been coined as a means of measuring and monitoring it. The proportion of births attended by skilled health personnel is an indicator included in the Millennium Development Goals. In recent years, however, global recognition of the difficulties and limitations in using this indicator has increased. What is needed to make "skilled attendants" provide skilled attendance (Graham, Bell, and Bullough 2001)? A health professional with a midwifery diploma will not necessarily make a difference if she does not have the needed skills, equipment, drugs, and help when things go wrong. Currently, no international consensus exists on how to design an indicator of maternal health care that would take account of all of these issues.

Care of Obstetric Emergencies and Complications

The skilled attendants who provide entry into the health system need to be complemented with the elements of care needed to manage the most common obstetric emergencies. Such care is classified in two tiers: basic essential obstetric care (bEOC) and comprehensive essential obstetric care (cEOC). Basic essential obstetric care, which is recommended for peripheral levels of the health care system, comprises treatment of severe infection by antibiotic injections, treatment of eclampsia with injectable anticonvulsants, intravenous infusion and injectables to treat postdelivery bleeding, assisted vaginal (complicated) delivery, and manual removal of the placenta. cEOC is recommended for central but commonly accessible levels of the health care system, such as the district hospital; in addition to the bEOC elements, it should include major surgery, blood transfusion, and care of pregnancy complications. UNICEF, WHO, and UNFPA (1997) defined the minimum density for provision of bEOC and cEOC as 4 units per 500,000 population for bEOC and 1 to 2 units per 500,000 population for cEOC.

How Best to Deliver Effective Interventions in Developing Countries?

No universal agreement exists on how best to deliver the critical elements of maternal health care in developing countries or on how to monitor its impact or cost. The earlier belief that training of traditional birth attendants (TBAs) would contribute greatly to MMR reduction has been disproved in recent years. Similarly, reliance on risk screening to determine which birthing women need professional care and which do not has lost credibility (Starrs 1998). Current information clearly indicates that care of obstetric emergencies needs to be accessible for all women because most complications are unpredictable and require prompt treatment. Today, development of such care is being given much emphasis (UNICEF, WHO, and UNFPA 1997). At the same time, experiences from a number of countries indicate that skilled attendance at all deliveries can be a major contributory factor in MMR reduction. These two strategies epitomize the main streams of current thought (Liljestrand 2000). The implicit policy question is: Should developing countries invest mainly in building capacity for dealing with obstetric emergencies, or in providing skilled attendance for all, with additional care for those who develop severe complications?

Research that could address such a question would be difficult to design, lengthy, and expensive. The case studies of Malaysia and Sri Lanka provide evidence that the two countries did not view the two strategies as competing alternatives. Instead, they moved stepwise and strategically to implement them as complementary strategies during the different phases of health care system development.

Aims of the Study

This study examines the chain of societal events leading to the continual strengthening of the health systems of Malaysia and Sri Lanka, the steps taken to strengthen maternal health care, and how each country and its communities afforded the steps.

The study addresses the following specific questions:

- *Supportive environment:* What were the main supportive factors in the environment leading to effective interventions in maternal health care?

- *Skilled attendance:*

  - How was a high proportion of skilled birth attendance achieved?

  - How was it made available to poor women and families?

  - What was the relationship between efforts to improve skilled birth attendance and care of obstetric emergencies?

  - How were these types of care made to interact?

- *Affordability:* How did these countries afford to improve maternal health?

- *Implementation:* How were the main bottlenecks resolved during different development periods?

Study Approach

The study uses a retrospective ecological approach and drew on quantitative and qualitative data.

Analysis of Quantitative and Qualitative Health Data

The study is based on the analysis of data from historical records and reports. The analysis is limited to periods of time for which data are available and accessible. Both countries have relatively strong systems of records of births and deaths, health service statistics, and basic economic data. Information on health services expenditures is limited and available mostly in an aggregate form. Sri Lankan statistical data on births and deaths, health, and fertility, as well as descriptive and analytical reports, are available for more than 90 years, but data on health services availability and utilization are limited. The equivalent Malaysian data and reports are available mainly for the post-Independence period. Prior to Malaysia's Independence in 1957, information was maintained separately for each state in the federation and was not accessible for this study. In both countries, the reliability of health service statistics has been validated previously by surveys (see chapters 2 and 3), and some estimates of the validity of death information are available.

The data for this study were supplemented by interviews with key informants who had personal experience in health and health-related systems in each country during key phases of development. Fourteen key informants in Malaysia and 14 in Sri Lanka were interviewed. In both countries, key informants included doctors, nurses, and midwives who had worked in small hospitals and in rural health services at both the district and the state or province level. They had subsequently become senior managers or clinicians at the national level. In addition, some key informants were economists who had studied the historical evolution of the social sector. A key informant in Sri Lanka was a former minister of health.

The interviews used a standardized guide and covered issues such as perceptions regarding key developmental landmarks; status of midwives during different time periods; the relationship between midwives, rural communities, and traditional birth attendants; incentives for staff to work in rural areas; obstetric practices; and payment for maternity services and training standards. The professional experiences of the key informants, in total, covered the period from the

1950s to date. Information from these interviews is cited as ([name], informant interview), and the informants are listed in Appendix 4.

Scope and Limitations of the Analysis

This study is an ecological analysis, which lacks the power of a planned, controlled trial that tests single interventions. The data encountered also did not provide substantial natural experiments, that is, data series comparing different states inside the countries. The data series were incomplete in that information for some years was missing. Nevertheless, this study constitutes the most complete analysis available of maternal health, maternal health care development, and health care expenditures in the two countries.

The analysis explores trends in the relationship between the percentage of women who had skilled attendance during childbirth and reductions in maternal mortality. It also examines the trends in the prevalence of skilled attendance at births among poor people and trends in public expenditures on health and on maternal health. The analysis focuses on how skilled attendance became widely prevalent even among the poor as well as on the affordability of such care.

The study developed evidence on improvements in other factors that are known to be related to maternal mortality, such as fertility, safe water and sanitation, and women's status. Insufficient data were available to support analyses that would have assessed the relative contribution of each of those factors.

Affordability: Assessment Approach

In light of the relative economic progress made by both countries, especially Malaysia, in recent decades, an obvious concern is the affordability of similar efforts in countries with lower incomes. Answering the question poses a number of methodological challenges. One critical issue in a study covering several decades is the change in the value of the national currencies over time due to inflation. Another predicament is posed by comparisons of the past efforts of Malaysia and Sri Lanka with those of other countries. Exchange rates used in foreign trade are not an appropriate basis for such comparisons because they do not accurately reflect the domestic purchasing power of the national currency in the acquisition of health service resources, which are labor intensive and mostly domestic in origin. The purchasing power parities of the currencies of the two countries, which could potentially address this problem, were not available for the entire period under study.

To address those issues and make the findings more universal, this study expresses both capital and operating expenditures in terms of their proportion to the total domestic resources available to the country at the relevant time period (that is, gross domestic product [GDP] at current prices). Specifically, for each year under study, annual data on total and maternal expenditures from each country were compared with GDP in current prices. The resulting expenditure data relative to GDP were then analyzed and compared over time and across countries.

Estimation of Expenditures versus Costing. This study relied on the estimation of expenditures rather than the estimation of costs for both conceptual and practical reasons. First, countries that need to embark on similar efforts should have the financial resources to undertake the task. For instance, a costing approach would have apportioned capital costs over the future life of assets acquired. However, countries would have needed to make the disbursement up front. Therefore, the costing approach would have underestimated the dimensions of the initial financial resources required, especially in an expanding system, and then overestimate capital outlays as the system matured. An important practical issue is that it was not possible to conduct a costing study of the services involved in the 1970s and 1980s because of the lack of relevant information.

Estimation and Uncertainty. This study has taken the approach that if the value of the estimates were to be misstated, it would be preferable to err on the high, rather than the low, side. Therefore, the estimates have attempted to include significant expenditures incurred throughout the two countries' ministries of health to ensure that the services were provided. When the basis of estimation was uncertain, an attempt was made to take the high side. Consequently, the estimates could be considered an upper limit of the expenditures that were actually incurred.

The Evidence

In the past 15 years, global awareness of the previously largely neglected challenge of maternal deaths has increased. Much more information has been gathered in recent years on the levels and causes of maternal mortality as well as on which interventions and main strategies work to reduce these deaths.

How Long Did It Take to Halve the Maternal Mortality Ratio?

More than a decade of experience with the Safe Motherhood initiatives with less than satisfactory progress has caused many developing countries, international agencies, and donors to wonder whether significant reduction of maternal mortality is possible within short periods of time. Was it realistic to aim for a 50 percent reduction of global MMR within the first 10 years after 1990, followed by a further 50 percent reduction during the next 15 years, by 2015, as indicated in the International Development Goals (IDGs)? The

Table 3. Amount of Time to Halve Maternal Mortality Ratio, Malaysia and Sri Lanka, 1949–92

	MMR*	
	MALAYSIA	SRI LANKA
3–7 years: introduction of modern medical advances into existing services	1950: 534 1957: 282	1947: 1,056 1950: 486
13 years: improved access for rural population	1957: 282 1970: 148	1950: 486 1963: 245
Every 6–12 years: quality improvement processes	1976: 78 1985: 37 1991: 18	1973: 121 1981: 58 1992: 27

*Maternal deaths per 100,000 live births.
Sources: Sri Lanka, Department of Census and Statistics, various years; Malaysia, Department of Statistics, various years.

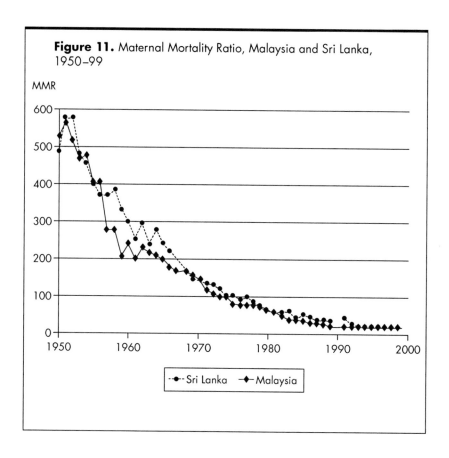

Figure 11. Maternal Mortality Ratio, Malaysia and Sri Lanka, 1950–99

Malaysian and Sri Lankan experiences indicate that the goals are achievable. Reductions in maternal mortality in both countries have been impressive (figure 11).

In both countries an initial period of rapid decline occurred, and MMR was reduced by half within 3 years (1947–50) in Sri Lanka and within 7 years (1950–57) in Malaysia (table 3). This dramatic fall in the MMR was probably associated with general health improvement, including malaria control, as well as the introduction of antibiotics and modern obstetric techniques to the sections of the population who had access to health care already. Prior to this period, however, both countries had established the foundations that enabled them to introduce modern obstetric care promptly and successfully. The critical elements of the foundation included establishment of systems to train and supervise midwives, regulate midwifery practices, and introduce accountability for results; systems for monitoring births and deaths; and models for effective communication with women and communities.

During the next period it took each country 13 years to slice MMR in half again. During this period it appears that critical elements of modern obstetric care were made accessible to the bulk of the rural population through development of a widespread rural health network. This network used trained, skilled midwives as its backbone along with hands-on support from supervisory staff competent in basic obstetrics and a system for prompt access to facilities that could treat obstetric complications.

During the subsequent decades, both Malaysia and Sri Lanka managed to reduce their MMR by 50 percent every 6 to 11 years using strategies aimed at increasing utilization of existing services through better management, a focus on quality, and systemic responsiveness to public needs and expectations.

Ensuring That Basic Services and Maternal Health Care Reach the Poor

The governments of Malaysia and Sri Lanka, backed by public sentiment, were almost revolutionary in their early identification of priority issues such as rights to equitable access to basic health services and education. Both countries regarded free health care for the poor as an essential element of national development, and they implemented specific, sustained human development strategies in health, education, and nutrition (Government of Malaysia, various years; Gunatilleke 2000). Both countries devoted special attention to providing geographical and financial access to education and health services for the rural poor, and both countries declared early that maternal and child health were national priorities. Both countries demonstrated sustained commitment for their priorities with financial, managerial, and political support. The countries were politically stable, and their political and management systems provided reasonably strong linkages and feedback between the rural poor and the ruling political establishment. In Sri Lanka, the political electoral system provided incentives for the political establishment to respond to the demands of the rural masses that formed the majority of the electorate. In Malaysia, the ethnic composition of the electorate provided political incentives to achieve better social and economic equity among different ethnic groups and states. Those pressures resulted in rapid and integrated rural development.

Thus, both countries made significant investments in expanding health services to rural areas during a relatively short period (10 to 15 years). Preventive health services and inpatient hospital care were financed largely through general taxation and were provided mainly by the public sector, whereas ambulatory medical care in urban areas was gradually provided to a greater extent by the private sector and financed by user fees. Maternity-related services—antenatal, childbirth, and postnatal care and child health services—were provided almost exclusively by the public sector until recently. Public health measures to improve sanitation and water supply and control of communicable diseases, particularly malaria, have been successful.

The impact of such policies is evident. Mortality of women of reproductive age has declined significantly during the period that is the subject of this study. The success of maternal health care interventions is evident from the large fall in the number of maternal deaths as a proportion of the total number of deaths among women of reproductive age—from about 10 percent to 1 percent, in the case of Malaysia. The fall was even larger in Sri Lanka, as discussed in the overview.

Moreover, strong evidence indicates that interventions reached the poor. For example, within a 20-year period in Malaysia, the group of states that had the highest household poverty rates managed to reduce their MMR to levels comparable to those of the states that had the lowest poverty rates (see figure 6 and chapter 2). Similarly, in Sri Lanka the disparity in MMR among different provinces was narrowed (see chapter 3).

Critical Strategies for Reducing Maternal Mortality Ratio

Three strategies emerge as critical elements in the approaches used in both countries:

1. Develop solid foundations to address maternal deaths, the building blocks of which consist of systems to

   • support professional midwifery,

   • monitor births and maternal deaths,

   • use maternal death information for high-profile advocacy, and

   • identify critical elements of locally successful models of care that can be replicated on a large scale.

2. Increase access to effective maternal care, particularly for the rural and the poor, by removing physical, social, and financial barriers and fostering community mobilization.

3. Improve utilization of available maternal health care services by raising quality through better clinical and organization management and empowerment of clients and communities.

The three strategies are interdependent. For example, improved access to maternal health care is effective only if frontline midwifery services are professionalized and linked to a health system that is able to respond promptly to emergencies and complications. Similarly, monitoring of maternal deaths is useful when it is used to fuel advocacy that is essential for sustained political and managerial commitment. Figure 12 summarizes the strategies and their interrelationships.

Health care systems capacity dictates the timing and implementation of each strategy. Pragmatism is needed in selecting the main focus of strategies for any particular phase of health systems development, and flexibility is required in adapting and expanding the implementation focus as health care systems' capacity improves. For example, during the 1950s and 1960s, Malaysia had low female literacy, and TBAs were an established feature in rural Malaysia. In this scenario, strategies that were successful in winning women to safer

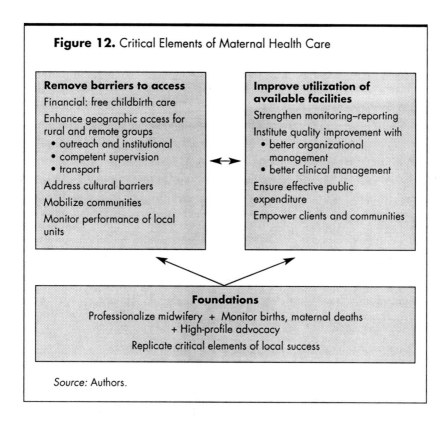

Figure 12. Critical Elements of Maternal Health Care

Remove barriers to access

Financial: free childbirth care

Enhance geographic access for rural and remote groups
- outreach and institutional
- competent supervision
- transport

Address cultural barriers

Mobilize communities

Monitor performance of local units

Improve utilization of available facilities

Strengthen monitoring–reporting

Institute quality improvement with
- better organizational management
- better clinical management

Ensure effective public expenditure

Empower clients and communities

Foundations

Professionalize midwifery + Monitor births, maternal deaths + High-profile advocacy

Replicate critical elements of local success

Source: Authors.

childbirth practices included building of partnerships with TBAs, as described in chapter 2. In the 1950s in Sri Lanka, however, TBAs were not prominent, and women were more literate than in Malaysia and wanted suitable facilities. Sri Lanka did not need to address an issue with TBAs, but it did need to respond to the strong demand for facilities that were easily accessible to remote areas. Sri Lanka provided small maternity homes in remote and rural areas, and women tended to seek admission to those facilities some time before delivery in order to have access to care in the event of complications.

Chapters 2 and 3 describe how Malaysia and Sri Lanka incrementally applied the strategies over four to five decades, during which time the capacity of the health care system gradually increased. This approach enabled the countries to achieve major gains, even when capacity was fairly weak, and to sustain continued decline of MMR even after achieving fairly low levels and in the face of the need for more stringent application of strategies.

Most of the strategies summarized in figure 12 are widely known; however, in many developing countries they are perceived to be difficult to implement. The Malaysian and Sri Lankan experience suggests that implementation is possible if the strategies are taken step by step, taking into consideration health system capacity and environmental forces. The next three sections elaborate on some critical elements often perceived as particularly difficult: improving access, providing skilled midwifery close to communities, and monitoring maternal deaths.

Improving Access

Some of the key implementation strategies for improving access to effective maternal health care when health systems capacity was weak in Malaysia and Sri Lanka were as follows:

- Relatively inexpensive, well-trained, government-employed midwives were rapidly deployed in a widespread network of community-based clinics and hospitals.

- Well-trained supervisory nurse–midwives or public health nurses were placed close to the frontline midwives, and they provided hands-on assistance during childbirth complications and organized referrals to suitable institutions.

- During child health clinics, antenatal clinics, and home visits, midwives provided sustained messages urging childbirth with skilled attendance.

- In Malaysia, partnerships were established between government midwives, nurse–midwives, and TBAs.

- Transportation (in Malaysia) or transportation subsidy (in Sri Lanka) was provided for sending emergencies to hospitals.

- In Malaysia, implementation of integrated rural development, which included coordinated investment in clinics, rural schools, and rural roads, was closely monitored with special attention to less developed states.

- In Sri Lanka, equitable social sector development was provided for all districts, including investment for free primary and secondary education, free health care, and food subsidies.

- Monitoring systems were strengthened to track implementation achievements and gaps.

- Special strategies for reaching out to the unreached and for mobilizing communities were developed.

The success of these strategies is evident. Within a decade it was possible to increase the proportion of women having childbirth with skilled attendance to more than 40 percent, and maternal mortality had been halved (table 4); although health systems' capacity was relatively weak, fertility was high, and female literacy comparatively low.

The Skilled Midwife as the Frontline Health Worker

The outstanding evolutionary feature of maternity-related health services in both countries is the pivotal role of trained and government-employed midwives. They have been relatively inexpensive to both countries, yet they have been the cornerstone for the expansion of an extensive health system to rural communities. They have provided accessible and culturally acceptable maternity services in hospitals and communities, gained sustained respect from the communities they serve, and are described with affection and admiration by managers and policymakers in each country (see boxes in chapters 2 and 3).

Critical features that characterize midwife services are technical competence acquired during a fairly short, basic training period, good supervision, and employment that offers financial and social security and manageable workloads. The basic training lasts 18 to 24 months and is oriented to clinical competence. The system of training and employment generates dedication and high morale. Midwives have become the frontline primary health care workers: for

Table 4. Key Health Features, Malaysia and Sri Lanka, 1940–61

	SRI LANKA		MALAYSIA	
	1940	1950	1952	1961
Maternal mortality ratio[a]	1,607	577	520	200
Childbirth				
Skilled attendance (%)	27	50+	+/– 30	41
In institutions (%)	—	36	+/– 18	25
Women's education and status				
Female literacy (%)	43.8[b]	54	17	32
Female-to-male literacy ratio (at the end of the period)	0.62[b]	0.71	0.32	0.47
Total fertility rate	—	5.0	—	6.0
Health service capacity				
Beds per 1,000 population	1.82[c]	2.6	2.5	2.4
Maternal and child health clinics (Malaysia) or health centers (Sri Lanka) per 100,000 live births	195	230	174	242[d]
Number of live births per obstetrician (public sector)	—	15,493	—	56,000[e]
Number of live births per trained midwife per year	218	158	461	320
Number of midwives and nurses per 100 government doctors	213	212	648	606
Population per doctor	14,782	10,529	8,728	6,500

— Not available.
[a] 11 percent are in small institutions.
[b] 1946 data.
[c] 1932 data.
[d] 1956 data.
[e] 1960 data.
Sources: Authors' compilation of data from various sources.

many people, midwives are the first point of contact with the formal health care system, both in terms of the care that they provide and the propelling of people further into the health system. It can be assumed that midwives' curative skills (such as suturing, stopping bleeding, diagnosing, and treating infection) enabled them to establish credibility during the initial stages and made the preventive and promotion work that they perform acceptable.

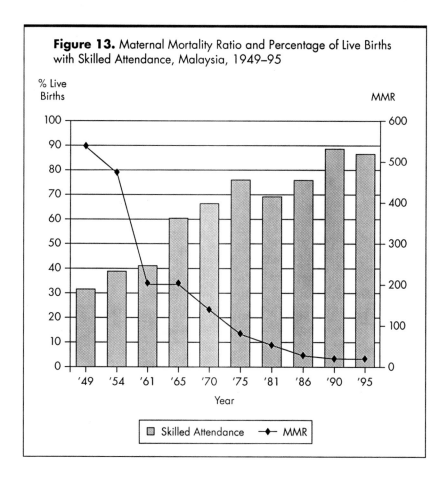

Figure 13. Maternal Mortality Ratio and Percentage of Live Births with Skilled Attendance, Malaysia, 1949–95

A review of the trends in births having skilled attendance and the decline in MMR shows that MMR decline began while skilled attendance was fairly low but increasing (figures 13 and 14). Clearly, midwives' hands-on skills were rapidly accepted and appreciated by communities in Malaysia and Sri Lanka. Even when only some of the women in a rural community actually used the services of the midwife, her presence was widely recognized and acknowledged, and she could be called upon during emergencies. This "momentum" effect—the awareness of the changing options due to the government's considerable efforts in the development of rural maternal and child health (MCH) care and the recent arrival of a skilled mid-

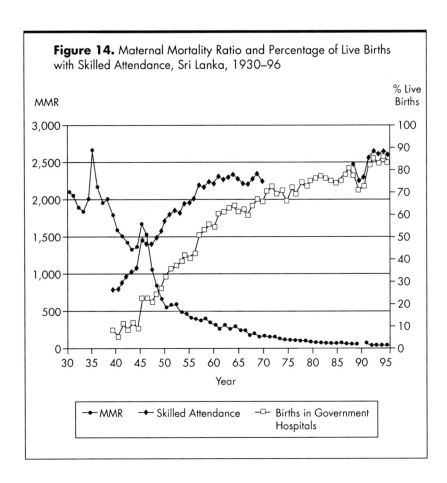

Figure 14. Maternal Mortality Ratio and Percentage of Live Births with Skilled Attendance, Sri Lanka, 1930–96

wife in the local community—partly explains why MMR fell drastically even when coverage of skilled birth attendance was comparatively low. This presence and impact is similar to that found in recent studies from Indonesia, where communities with a functioning "village midwife" (*bidan di desa*) have a lower incidence of low birth weight and malnutrition in general (Frankenberg and Thomas 2001).[3]

Better Data for Advocacy, Planning, and Monitoring

Better information on maternal deaths and imaginative use of such information is the key to building and sustaining political and community-level commitment and to improving the performance of the health system. These case studies demonstrate how three sources of such information can be used, progressively strengthened, and inter-linked. Civil registration of births and deaths, which had been established primarily for reasons unrelated to health care, provided analytic reports on maternal deaths. When the civil system was relatively weak, information was supplemented by efforts of local health staff, who sought information on maternal deaths through community sources, including local TBAs. Health service information systems, including hospital and medical records, provided increasingly sophisticated information on the numbers and causes of maternal deaths. Special systems were established for investigating factors contributing to maternal deaths; those systems involved communities, outreach health workers, TBAs, clinical staff in health centers and hospitals, and high-level managers at the district and national levels. Information from each of these sources has been consistently used to focus attention on maternal deaths and to monitor progress at district and institutional levels.

Maternal Mortality Transition: A Model for Action

From the evolutionary experience of Malaysia and Sri Lanka, a maternal mortality transition model emerges that provides a basis for other countries to analyze current situations and select priority policies and actions (figure 15). The transition model presents four developmental phases, which are characterized by the level of MMR and the percentage of births with skilled attendance. Each phase merges gradually into the next. The phases are associated with a changing profile of maternal deaths, which, taken in concert with existing health service capacity, education and female literacy, and women's status, provides pointers for immediate priority action.

During the earliest phase, MMR is high, health system capacity is weak, and skilled attendance is low. The priority is on advocacy to raise awareness of the seriousness and implications of high maternal mortality, efforts that are supported through maternal death infor-

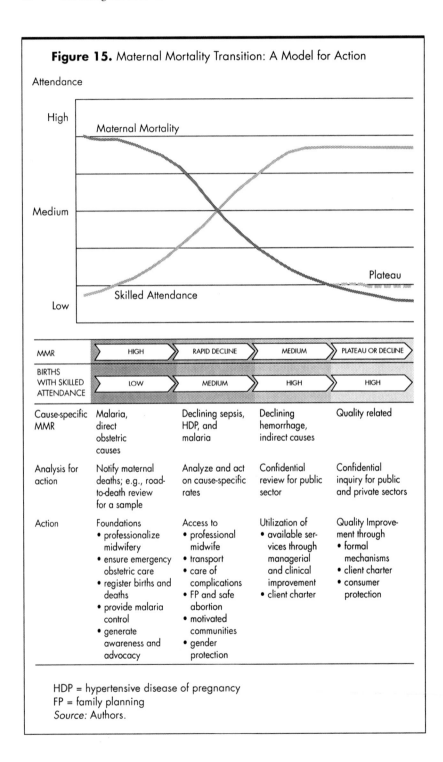

Figure 15. Maternal Mortality Transition: A Model for Action

MMR	HIGH	RAPID DECLINE	MEDIUM	PLATEAU OR DECLINE
BIRTHS WITH SKILLED ATTENDANCE	LOW	MEDIUM	HIGH	HIGH
Cause-specific MMR	Malaria, direct obstetric causes	Declining sepsis, HDP, and malaria	Declining hemorrhage, indirect causes	Quality related
Analysis for action	Notify maternal deaths; e.g., road-to-death review for a sample	Analyze and act on cause-specific rates	Confidential review for public sector	Confidential inquiry for public and private sectors
Action	Foundations • professionalize midwifery • ensure emergency obstetric care • register births and deaths • provide malaria control • generate awareness and advocacy	Access to • professional midwife • transport • care of complications • FP and safe abortion • motivated communities • gender protection	Utilization of • available services through managerial and clinical improvement • client charter	Quality Improvement through • formal mechanisms • client charter • consumer protection

HDP = hypertensive disease of pregnancy
FP = family planning
Source: Authors.

mation from civil registration and hospital-based reports. Midwifery could be professionalized through legislation, agreement on essential competencies for midwives and feasible training modalities, and certification and registration of midwives following recognized training. Addressing major disease problems, such as malaria and malnutrition, also produces gains in maternal health. Local models of maternal health care found to be effective in small areas could be analyzed to identify critical elements that would need to be included in large-scale replication. For example, in Malaysia, MCH clinic and outreach services that were found to be popular in urban and periurban Local Authority[4] settings were later replicated in rural areas. Similarly, in Sri Lanka, when it was found that districts that had Health Units[5] performed better during the disastrous nationwide malaria epidemic than districts that had no Health Units, the policy was adopted to extend Health Units to all districts.

During the next phase of health systems development, system capacity begins to improve as services become accessible to larger proportions of the population. MMR begins to decline rapidly, even when skilled attendance is fairly low (40 percent to 50 percent). Maternal deaths due to sepsis decline. The priority for policies and programs is to increase accessibility to essential maternal health care for the poor and rural segments of the population. In addition to access to competent, skilled midwives, services to treat pregnancy complications need to be upgraded and systems to facilitate prompt handling of emergencies need to be implemented. Communities need to be mobilized to recognize and respond to emergencies in childbirth. The impact of such measures can be monitored in the changing profile of maternal deaths: deaths due to infections and obstructed labor decrease, and deaths due to hemorrhage begin to decline.

Once the health service network has achieved fairly high geographic coverage, priority shifts to measures that aim to improve utilization of available services. For example, quality of care must be improved through strengthened clinical and organizational management measures. Quality improvement incentives and mechanisms need to encompass all types of private and public providers. Information, education, and feedback mechanisms that empower clients also are required. Institutional facilities for childbirth probably need to be expanded and strengthened as demand increases. As access to blood transfusions and institutions improves, deaths from hemorrhage decline.

Monitoring and modalities for investigation of maternal deaths must be modified in accordance with the numbers of deaths that occur and the capacity of the system to implement investigations into factors contributing to deaths. When the health system is relatively weak and maternal deaths are numerous, feasibility might be limited to the investigation of a sample of deaths, followed by high-profile action aimed at correcting systemic weaknesses and mobilizing commitment for action and resources. When capacity strengthens and deaths decline, sophisticated investigations and analysis, such as those implemented in more industrialized countries, become possible. In either circumstance, the critical element is the proactive use of data for priority actions and advocacy.

In most developing countries, it is likely that different parts of the country are at different phases in the MMR transition model. For example, urban areas and industrialized districts might have fairly high geographic coverage of services, whereas the urban poor and less developed districts might have poor access. Thus, different priorities apply to different situations. Subnational analysis and pragmatic selection and implementation of activities are keys to success. The experiences of Malaysia and Sri Lanka illustrate the adaptation of national programs to local needs. In the 1980s, Sri Lanka identified poor maternal health in the ethnic Indian population on estates and developed specific strategies to improve Indians' access to and utilization of services. Similarly, when health system capacity was weak in the less developed states in Malaysia, nurse–midwives were empowered to perform clinical life-saving interventions that were performed only by doctors in other states.

Countries need to assess their current status and select policy options that are feasible and most likely to provide immediate impact within their own context. For example, in many countries today, pregnant women face financial barriers when they experience complications in pregnancy either because they are uninsured or because formal and informal charges[6] for health are beyond their means. Some countries have worked hard to improve access for rural women, but rural women often are reluctant to use the available services because midwives do not have the clinical skills or the drugs and equipment to deal with complications. Similarly, institutional services to deal with complications are underdeveloped or inaccessible. Single interventions are unlikely to be effective. Appropriately selected packages of interventions are critical for success.

Fertility Decline and Maternal Mortality

This study did not have sufficiently detailed data on fertility at successive points in time to assess the relative contribution of changes in fertility to maternal mortality decline. However, it has been possible to review trends in fertility compared with MMR.

No significant decline in the total fertility rate (TFR)—the average number of children that a woman age 15 can expect to bear if she lives until at least age 50—has been found for either country before 1960. In other words, fertility was largely unchecked by contraception before that year and fertility decline thus had little impact on the steep MMR decline of the 1950s. Since the 1960s, both countries have experienced major declines in fertility, and since 1960 the TFR decline has had a stable association with MMR decline. The fall of TFR has been largest in Sri Lanka, which now has fertility at population replacement level (TFR was 5 in 1960 and is now around 2), but the decline has also been substantial in Malaysia (whose TFR was 6.3 in 1960 and is 3.3 today; see figures 16 and 17). In Sri Lanka, the age of marriage and first birth have also been rising over recent decades. Family planning has been an integral component of MCH services since the 1970s in both countries. Clearly, family planning and falling fertility have contributed to the reduction of maternal deaths in both countries, through both preventing unwanted pregnancies and reducing high-risk pregnancies at the upper ends of the age spectrum and among the very young. The problem of maternal deaths due to unsafe abortion also has been gradually dealt with in

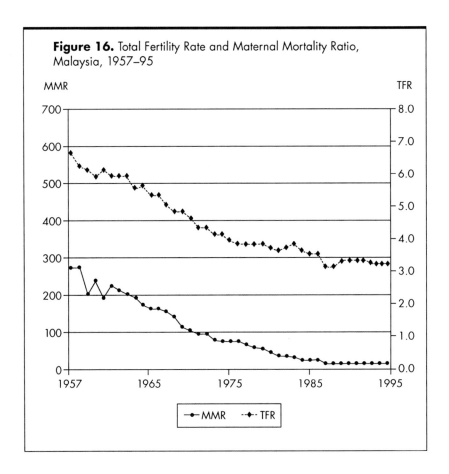

Figure 16. Total Fertility Rate and Maternal Mortality Ratio, Malaysia, 1957–95

both countries, partly through better access to family planning. Moreover, it can be expected that when a health system provides credible and attractive basic services in key areas of women's health (that is, maternal health care and contraceptive care), those services will reinforce each other. Maternal mortality and fertility declines are thus interwoven through increased uptake of both services.

The initial steep fall in the MMR happened without notable TFR decline, whereas after 1960 maternal deaths were prevented in Malaysia and Sri Lanka as a result of declines in fertility. The concomitant investment in women's education and health, maternal health care, and family planning have, with all probability, con-

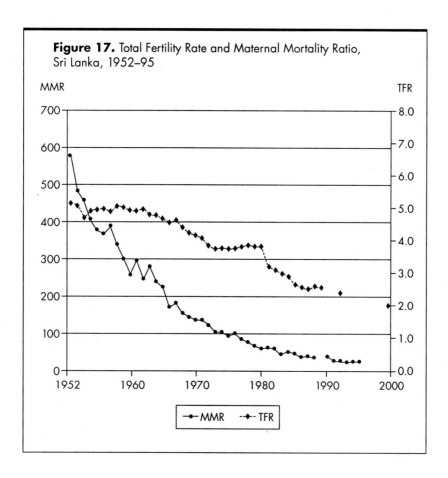

Figure 17. Total Fertility Rate and Maternal Mortality Ratio, Sri Lanka, 1952–95

tributed greatly to the synergies among the interventions in health, maternal health, and fertility.

Newborn Survival and Maternal Health

Although the focus of this study is on maternal health, it is useful to look briefly at the simultaneous improvements in newborn[7] health and survival. The determinants of maternal and newborn health overlap to a large extent in that interventions to save mothers' lives also improve outcomes of newborns, particularly during the early newborn period. About two-thirds of newborn deaths take place in the first week, and two-thirds of those deaths take place in the first day after birth (Save the Children USA 2001). Later deaths among infants may be less dependent on maternal health care and more dependent on factors such as water, sanitation, and breastfeeding practices. It should also be remembered that deaths during the first week of life are roughly equal to the rate of stillbirths. For example, if 2 percent of newborns die during the first week of life, the rate of stillbirth is about 2 percent. Stillborns are often not counted, and information is often shaky on the national level in many developing countries, but other studies have demonstrated this to be the case. Consequently, when we reduce newborn deaths, we also reduce stillbirths.

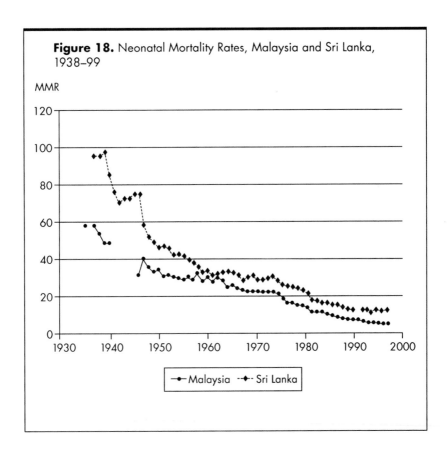

Figure 18. Neonatal Mortality Rates, Malaysia and Sri Lanka, 1938–99

The declines in newborn deaths have been progressive over the decades studied and have a similar steep initial decline to that of MMR (figure 18). For instance, in Malaysia reductions in the neonatal mortality rate have continued in every decade since the 1950s. This pattern reflects the fact that basic newborn health care is largely provided in tandem with maternal health care. After a certain stage, however, newborn mortality may not follow MMR. Further reductions in mortality among the newborn may demand specific services or a higher level of quality. The initial decline of newborn deaths depends on the improved health of mothers and better maternal health services. Later falls in newborn deaths will require more sophisticated newborn health services.

This study also does not address morbidity of newborns or mothers. One aspect of newborn morbidity is reflected in rates of low birth weight. It is of concern that in Sri Lanka the rate of low birth weight has remained high for a long period, averaging around 25 percent and most recently (1999) estimated at 16.4 percent. The complex and important challenges of low birth weight and its evolution in these countries is not covered in this study.

Affordability of Public Expenditures on Health and Maternal and Child Health Care

Maternal health care in both countries has been provided largely by the public sector. This study examines two aspects of affordability. First, how did the countries afford it? Second, how could the clients, particularly the poor, afford to use maternal health care?

Analysis shows that total public expenditures on health care have been modest, amounting to only about 1.4 percent to 1.8 percent of GDP in Malaysia and an average of 1.8 percent of GDP in Sri Lanka (table 5). In Malaysia, expenditures on maternal health care in public hospitals and MCH services in the community were only 0.38 percent of GDP, on average; in Sri Lanka, expenditures were even lower, at 0.23 percent of GDP. Note that Sri Lanka completed its initial investment in building its extensive health infrastructure of clinics and hospitals in rural areas prior to the 1950s, whereas

Table 5. Public Expenditures on Health Services and Maternal Health Care, Malaysia and Sri Lanka, 1950s–90s

	MALAYSIA				SRI LANKA			
	TOTAL HEALTH SERVICES	MATERNAL HEALTH CARE (% OF GDP)			TOTAL HEALTH SERVICES	MATERNAL HEALTH CARE (% OF GDP)		
PERIOD		CAPITAL	OPERATING	TOTAL		CAPITAL	OPERATING	TOTAL
1950–55	—	—	—	—	1.71	0.03	0.24	0.28
1956–60	1.54	—	—	—	2.29	0.04	0.24	0.28
1961–65	1.71	—	—	—	2.11	0.03	0.27	0.31
1966–70	—	—	—	—	2.10	0.03	0.26	0.29
1971–75	1.79	0.06	0.26	0.32	1.81	0.04	0.23	0.28
1976–80	1.63	0.05	0.31	0.36	1.62	0.04	0.19	0.23
1981–85	1.59	0.08	0.33	0.41	1.30	0.03	0.13	0.16
1986–90	1.51	0.06	0.34	0.40	1.72	0.06	0.13	0.19
1991–95	1.44	0.05	0.32	0.37	1.52	0.03	0.13	0.17
1996–99	n.a.	n.a.	n.a.	n.a.	1.56	0.03	0.10	0.14
1950–99	—	—	—	—	1.79	0.04	0.20	0.23

n.a. Not applicable.
Note: Maternal health care data include hospital care for deliveries and complications of pregnancy and community-based maternal and child health care services. Data may not sum to totals due to rounding.

Malaysia's rural health service was developed and hospitals were upgraded and expanded after Independence in 1957.

Although the two countries were poorer than they are today and had different levels of GDP per capita in the 1960s and 1970s, it is remarkable that both countries were spending 0.28 to 0.34 percent of GDP on maternal child health care funded from the public purse. It is also relevant to note that the levels of capital expenditures that reflect market prices of construction and equipment remained relatively stable during the period under review. Operating expenses, however, which mirror the number and salary rates of public servants, show a declining trend in the case of Sri Lanka and a later, smaller decline in Malaysia. This decrease was achieved despite the increasing numbers of health professionals employed. The lowering of salary rates of health professionals in relation to GDP per capita allowed the engagement of a greater number of public servants without a proportional increase in operating expenditures.

Removing Financial Barriers for Clients

Public sector health services are financed through general taxation and are free to the poor and mostly free to other people in both countries. Successive governments in each country adopted policies to remove possible financial barriers to the use of maternal health care during pregnancy and childbirth. Household surveys, as well as interviews of key informants in Malaysia, confirm that personal preventive services, such as antenatal care, have been free. In general, public sector ambulatory care is free or practically free (less than US$0.30 per visit), and more than half of those hospitalized for any reason (other than maternal) in a government facility pay less than US$3 per admission. In Sri Lanka, review of administrative reports, including revenues collected, user fee policies, and interviews with key informants, confirms that services associated with maternal health services are practically free to the client. Furthermore, similar proportions of women from low- and high-income groups (70 percent to 80 percent) use public sector hospitals for childbirth.

Conclusion

The main findings of the study demonstrate how the rapid reduction of maternal mortality can occur when systematic placement of rural midwives leads to increased access to maternal health care, including referral care for severe complications. The foundations for such improvements are government commitment to poverty reduction and equity as well as the formal recognition and support of midwifery and registration of births and deaths. Continual momentum over the decades for seeking pragmatic and affordable solutions to improving maternal health was provided by the continual analysis of the circumstances of individual maternal deaths. In the period of analysis, public expenditures on maternal health care initially constituted one-fifth of the total public expenditures on health, which at that time totaled 1.8 percent of GDP for both countries in 1971–75. Since then, public expenditures on health care as a proportion of GDP in the two countries have declined; the proportion of GDP spent on maternal health care has declined considerably in Sri Lanka, but not in Malaysia until recently. Maternal health care throughout the period has been free or almost free to clients, and emergency transportation has been subsidized.

A somewhat surprising conclusion suggested by this study contributes to the current global debate as to whether skilled attendance at birth or the care of obstetric emergencies is the most important approach to reducing maternal mortality in developing countries. The answer appears to be that the presence of a respected and skilled birth attendant (that is, midwife) in the village or the vicinity, backed by facilities providing care of obstetric emergencies, is an effective way to reach women with basic maternal health care. In doing so, even with skilled birth attendance at only 40 to 50 percent of all births, the majority of the population can have access to essential care and MMR can be reduced to fewer than 200 maternal deaths per 100,000 live births.

An "MMR transition model for action" emerges from analysis of the implementation experience of Sri Lanka and Malaysia. It provides pointers for policies and actions for countries that are at different phases of health care systems development. Different regions within a country might be in different phases of health care systems development, and different groups within a country might face different barriers to care. As a result, some countries might need to implement different sets of policies and priority actions simultaneously to meet the challenges of "double phases" within a country.

At a time when many developing countries are struggling to simultaneously balance national budgets and reduce poverty, the main message from this study is that consistent prioritization and investment in basic health services and in critical elements of maternal health care have an impact at a relatively low level of expenditure. Reducing maternal mortality has been variously seen as a difficult "nut to crack" as well as "the scandal of our time"—but it can be done.

optimistic outlook

Maternal health care needs to be part of a development strategy that includes poverty reduction and other basic services, such as water and sanitation, malaria control, nutrition, and empowerment and education of women. Access to maternal health care can be increased gradually, if it is based on popular involvement and continual reviews of maternal deaths. The elimination of financial barriers to care and the provision of subsidies for emergency transportation make an essential contribution. The maintenance and improvement of high-quality maternal health care require an ongoing effort that will have different emphases at different phases of health systems development. But in all phases, commitment to health of the most vulnerable groups—mothers and children—is essential. Sustained commitment of modest financial investments and effective implementation of policy options can enable countries to achieve the Millennium Development Goals for maternal health.

Notes

1. Skilled attendance refers to deliveries by clinically trained midwives, nurse–midwives, or doctors. The actual services provided include prenatal and postnatal care.

2. The lifetime risk of maternal mortality in a given country is the risk for a woman in that country to die a maternal death during her lifetime. Lifetime risk depends on the risk of a maternal death, once pregnant, and the average fertility in the country.

3. The training of 72,000 *bidan di desa* in Indonesia during the 1990s has received mixed reviews and still faces the challenge of full consolidation. Access to maternal health care has increased for rural populations, and the quality of care (leading to higher use and credibility) has improved with standards, retraining, and supervision. The sustainability issues are currently being addressed.

4. "Local Authorities" are semi-autonomous municipalities and town councils.

5. The Health Unit system provides health prevention and promotion services at the community level by a medical officer and a team of field health workers

6. Informal charges are payments made when no official fees are set but payment is required by custom or demanded by the provider unofficially.

7. In this context the newborn period refers to the first 4 weeks of life.

CHAPTER 2

Malaysia

Background: Malaysia Today

Malaysia is situated in the heart of Southeast Asia and is a federation of 13 states. It has a multiparty political system with democratically elected state assemblies and a federal parliament. The prime minister is a member of the majority party in the federal parliament and is appointed by the king. It is an ethnically diverse country (ethnic Malays, 58 percent; ethnic Chinese, 24 percent; ethnic Indians, 7 percent; and the remaining 11 percent are made up of Aboriginals, Indonesians, Filipinos, Eurasians, Europeans, and others). Malaysia's administrative, legal, political, educational, and health systems were established during more than a century of British colonial rule and were patterned on British models. Table 6 presents basic information about the country.

The Malaysian public health care system consists of an extensive network of clinics and hospitals and preventive health services funded through general taxation. The services are highly subsidized and are mostly free to clients. Household surveys indicate that 50 to 80 percent of respondents who have used a public sector facility for ambulatory care reported that it was free or practically free (less than RM1 per visit, or US$0.30 equivalent). Half of those hospitalized in a government facility paid less than RM13 (about US$3 per admission). The public health system is well utilized and accounts for 78 percent of hospitalization and 43 percent of ambulatory care for ill-

Table 6. Malaysia at a Glance

	1957	1995
Infant mortality per 1,000 live births	75	9
Life expectancy (years)	57	72
Maternal mortality per 100,000 live births	282	20
Total fertility rate	6.7	3.4
RECENT DATA		
Annual population growth rate (%)		2.4
Female literacy rate (%)[a]		70
GNP per capita[b]		US$3,400
GNP per capita growth rate (1998–99)		1.9
Households below the poverty line (%)[b]		8
Male-to-female literacy ratio[a]		1.07:1
Population (millions)		23
Population in urban areas (%)		62
Population living within 3 km of a health facility (%)[a]		86
Population with access to safe drinking water (%)[a]		90
Population with access to sanitation (%)[a]		97
Population younger than age 20 (%)		45
Skilled attendance at childbirth (%)[a]		96
Total health expenditures (% of gross domestic product)[a]		2.4

GNP = Gross national product.
[a]1997 data.
[b]1999 data.
Sources: Authors' compilation of data from various sources.

ness. Personal preventive services, such as prenatal care and immunization, are obtained largely from public sector services. A smaller, urban-oriented web of private sector, largely for-profit clinics and hospitals provides mainly curative care and is financed largely through user fees. Payments for health care in both the public and the private sectors are largely made by users (64 percent) or employers (16 percent; Public Health Institute 1988, 1997).

Political Context

The territory of the Malay Peninsula, together with Singapore, fell progressively under British rule over 150 years during the 19th and 20th centuries. In 1957, Malaya became an independent nation consisting of a federation of 11 states in the Malay Peninsula. During the decades of British colonial rule, an active economy was established. However, economic activity was concentrated in the western coastal states. At that time the Malay population was involved mainly in rural agricultural pursuits and British policies encouraged the migration of workers from China and India to support the economic development of the territory. The socioeconomic development of the three major ethnic groups evolved at different paces, as did their health status and utilization of health services. For many years, ethnic Malays remained largely rural agricultural workers, ethnic Chinese were active in tin mines and urban commercial activities, and ethnic Indians worked mainly as indentured labor on rubber estates (Kennedy 1993).

World War II brought occupation by Japanese military forces from 1942 to 1945, which caused severe economic and social disruption, but the country recovered rapidly. An internal, communist-inspired insurgency (known as the Emergency) began in 1948 and led to large-scale resettlement of rural Chinese into so-called new villages. The Emergency increased the urbanization of the ethnic Chinese population. By 1950, with the Korean War boom, the economy had recovered from the disruption of WWII and was set on a course of expansion (IBRD 1955).

In 1957, the new nation of Malaya had an ethnically diverse population with significant differences in socioeconomic status among the ethnic groups. The population was more than 60 percent rural, and the 11 component states were vastly dissimilar in terms of economic development and ethnic composition. Independence stimulated nation-building efforts and gave a sense of belonging to all states in the new federation. Social and economic development initiatives were specifically targeted to the rural population and the less developed states, and implementation was closely monitored.

In 1963, Singapore and two states on the island of Borneo (Sarawak and Sabah) joined the federation, but Singapore left in 1965. When Sarawak and Sabah joined the federation, they were less developed than the peninsular states, and this lag was also evident in their health status. Data for Sarawak and Sabah are patchy; therefore, the analysis for this study, with the exception of the health expenditure analysis, is confined to Peninsular Malaysia.

Initially, modern medicine was introduced to colonial Malaya in the form of hospitals and public health measures, such as sanitation, water supply, and malaria control, to serve mainly the colonial officers and their families in urban areas. High death rates among the imported labor force caused growing interest and led to the extension of basic health services, including malaria control, sanitation, and medical care, to areas in which the immigrant labor population was concentrated. During the early years of the 20th century, as female migration increased, concern grew over high infant and maternal mortality among migrants. In addition, sociopolitical movements in Britain raised awareness of these health issues among the colonial administrators (Manderson 1996).

As a result, maternity-related services were introduced in hospitals and in urban and periurban communities in colonial Malaya. The community-based services (described later in this chapter) were designed on the pattern of the British district health nursing service (Manderson 1996; Phua 1987). Maternal mortality began to decline in the 1930s, when the maternal mortality ratio (MMR) was reported to be greater than 1,100 maternal deaths per 100,000 live births. The rate of decline accelerated after World War II and continued on a spectacular fall to about 20 deaths per 100,000 live births by 1990.

This study examines the improvement in maternal health from 1946–95 in the context of the historical development of the health system. It has a special focus on skilled attendance[1] during childbirth and the socioeconomic and political environment that enabled growth in skilled attendance. Particular attention is devoted to the affordability of maternal health care.

Study Approach

Several previous studies have described and commented on selected aspects of the Malaysian experience in reducing maternal mortality. Manderson (1996) and Phua (1987) discussed health systems development prior to Independence. Raj Karim (2000) described the major Safe Motherhood interventions implemented mainly during the 1980s and 1990s, and Koblinski, Campbell, and Heichelheim (1999) analyzed the model demonstrated by the Malaysian maternal health care system. This study expands on previous descriptions and analyses; it is the first of its kind to present trends in MMR and use of skilled attendance at birth and to analyze related health care systems policies, programs, expenditures, and capacity. This chapter also describes policies and programs in related sectors that provided a supportive environment for improvements in MMR.

Maternal Mortality Data Availability and Quality

Malaysia has a fairly comprehensive system of reporting births and deaths; they are reported at local police stations and are the peripheral sources of data for the registrar general (RG). During the period under study, the actual MMR was probably higher than the reported ratio because of underreporting of maternal deaths (see Appendix 1). Data on causes of maternal deaths throughout the study period are inadequate for deriving trends that can support conclusions. The system of birth registration has been in place since the early 1900s, but live births were grossly underreported until the early 1950s, when the National Registration System (NRS) was implemented. Introduced as a security measure during the Emergency, the identity card provided by the NRS became the basis for individual participation in the social and economic life of the country. Because the issuance of the identity card was based on the birth certificate, both civil and political authorities made strenuous efforts to improve birth registration, and reporting probably improved substantially.

During the 1950s and 1960s causes of maternal death were recorded only for deaths that occurred after the patient entered the hospital. At that time only about 30 percent of births had skilled attendance, and the cause of death was known for about 50 percent of reported maternal deaths. Even in 1998 only 44 percent of all deaths were medically certified. Maternal deaths accounted for about 10 percent of reported deaths among women of reproductive age from 1957–70. They continued to fall to about 6 percent in the 1970s and reached 2 percent by 1991. During the 1970s, government midwives working in rural areas instituted a practice of visiting families who reported female deaths to the local RG to assess whether it was a maternal death and determine the factors contributing to the death. During the next two decades, the system was expanded and strengthened, and by the early 1980s the Ministry of Health (MOH) was aware of more deaths associated with pregnancy and childbirth than the RG's count. The RG continued to be the official source of data on maternal deaths, however, and all official records use the RG data. Not until the early 1990s was the RG's system revised to take into account the deaths known to the MOH; this change could partially explain the recorded slowing of MMR decline in the 1990s.

Quality of Health Services and Utilization Data

Although rich descriptive information about the development of the health system and its sociopolitical environment is available for a 70-year period from 1930 onward, statistical data on health services and their utilization is fragmented among various state territories and local authorities and has many gaps and uncertainties (Government of Malaya 1936, 1939; Federation of Malaya various years).

Before Independence each of the component states in Malaya had its own health management system, and health system information was not standardized or collated to cover all 13 states that eventually became Malaysia. Urban Local Authorities—the local governments of the larger cities, such as Kuala Lumpur and George Town—provided most community-based services related to maternal health and maintained their own records. State governments maintained hospital data; private sector data were not collected. Although information systems improved from 1957–79, some major data gaps exist for health services and their utilization during the 1970s, and information from Urban Local Authorities and the private sector was not standardized with that of the MOH. After 1980, the MOH standardized the monitoring system nationwide; this improvement included the public and private sectors, and information generated by the system compares well with data obtained through nationwide household sample surveys (Public Health Institute 1988, 1997). Again, this study does not include Sarawak and Sabah, which joined Malaysia at a later stage and had information systems that lagged.

Expenditure Data on Health Services and Maternal Health Care

Details on the approach, methods, and sources used in estimating maternal health care (and some preventive child health care) expenditures are provided in Appendix 1. The estimates of public sector expenditures on health services cover the period from 1946–95. The estimates include capital and operational expenditures on preventive and curative services provided in institutional and community settings by local and central governments. Data gaps exist especially for the period 1966–70.

In this study, estimation of expenditures on maternal health care attendance is limited to the period 1971–95 because of missing data for earlier periods. Therefore, that analysis begins at a time when considerable coverage of the rural population had been achieved. Estimates include capital and operating expenditures for maternal and child health (MCH) clinic and outreach services in the community and for maternity services in public sector hospitals, including the teaching hospitals under the Ministry of Education (see Appendix 1). Estimates of operating expenses include expenditures on training, administration related to maternity and child health services, and related supplies and pharmaceuticals. Basic training of doctors undertaken by the Ministry of Education is not included. Five-year aggregates are used to show trends more clearly and to avoid some fluctuations that occurred in single years as a result of large increases in salaries of public servants and the lumpy nature of investments in hospital facilities. Estimates are based on assumptions that would place the estimates on the high side of the band of uncertainty, and the analysis may overestimate operating expenditures related to skilled attendance by as much as 10 to 15 percent. The out-of-pocket expenditure data were obtained from two national household sample surveys conducted in 1986–87 and 1996–97 (Public Health Institute 1988, 1997).

Decline in Maternal Mortality

The decline in maternal mortality has been spectacular and sustained. During the 64-year period from 1933–97, the time taken to halve maternal mortality has been between 6 and 13 years, except for the initial period, which took 17 years, and the most recent period (after 1990), when MMR seems to have plateaued (table 7).

This chapter addresses four critical themes. First, it describes how maternal mortality declined among the disadvantaged groups in the population, an indication that efforts to improve access were successful. Second, it traces trends in the availability and use of skilled attendants and institutional childbirth against a background of maternal mortality decline. Third, it presents an analysis of key policy and program interventions to make childbearing safer during the successive phases of health systems development and describes critical policies in related sectors that enabled those interventions.

Table 7. Amount of Time to Halve the Maternal Mortality Ratio, Peninsular Malaysia, 1933–97

YEAR	MMR[a]	INTERVAL YEARS
1933	1,085	n.a.
1950	534	17
1957	282	7
1970	148	12
1976	78	6
1985	37	9
1991	18	6
1997	19	6[b]

n.a. Not applicable.
[a]Maternal deaths were probably underreported this entire time, although reporting did improve after the mid-1970s. By the mid-1990s, evidence indicated that actual MMRs were probably twice the official figures given in this table.
[b]No significant reduction in MMR.
Source: Malaysia, Department of Statistics, 1991; and Malaysia, Ministry of Health, various years.

Fourth, it explores the affordability of MMR reduction through analysis of public expenditures on health services for maternal health care. It also examines the affordability of those services to families.

Benefits for Developing Sectors of Society

Deliberate government policies and their consistent implementation, as described later in this chapter, ensured that disadvantaged groups benefited from health and social sector programs. The success of such efforts is evident in the comparative decline in maternal mortality in different ethnic groups and in the different component states in Malaysia.

Narrowing the Interethnic Gap. The urban ethnic Chinese have experienced better economic status and lower maternal mortality than have ethnic Malays and ethnic Indians. During the period 1957–95, however, MMR declined rapidly among all ethnic groups and the MMR gap between ethnic groups narrowed. For example, in 1957 ethnic Malays had 259 more maternal deaths per 100,000 live births than ethnic Chinese. By 1990, ethnic Malays had only 16 more deaths per 100,000 live births than ethnic Chinese (table 8).

Eliminating the Interstate Gap. Four peninsular states—Kelantan, Kedah, Perlis, and Terengganu—are rural and have been designated

Table 8. Maternal Mortality Ratio, by Ethnic Group, Peninsular Malaysia, 1957–90

YEAR	MMR			
	MALAYS	CHINESE	INDIANS	AVERAGE FOR ALL ETHNIC GROUPS
1957	399	140	205	282
1962	365	62	112	230
1967	259	49	99	168
1972	160	25	79	107
1977	113	21	52	79
1982	71	11	25	51
1985	48	13	20	37
1990	25	9	15	20

Source: Malaysia, Department of Statistics, 1991; and Malaysia, Ministry of Health, various years.

by the Economic Planning Unit of the Prime Minister's Department as "less developed." They have had higher poverty levels than the "more developed" states. For example, in 1997 the proportion of households below the poverty line in the less developed states was between 11 and 19 percent, whereas in other states the proportion ranged from 1 to 5 percent (Government of Malaysia 2000). The 1960s and 1970s brought efforts to improve access to health care for the rural poor, and poverty reduction efforts began in 1970 (Fadil 1997).

Prior to the 1970s, MMR in the less developed states was more than twice that of the more developed states. By 1990, the less developed states had caught up with the more developed states in terms of MMR (see figure 6 in the Overview), although a poverty gap remained. Poor people have benefited in an equitable way from the development of maternity-related services.

Skilled Attendance at Birth

During the 50-year period between 1945 and 1995, the proportion of live births with skilled attendance increased dramatically, from about 30 percent in 1949 to more than 90 percent in 1995 (figure 19 and table 9).

At the beginning of the period under study, maternal health services were largely urban and were provided through MCH clinics and hospitals. During the initial period (1945–56), the growth in skilled attendance (from 32 percent in 1949 to 39 percent in 1956) was due mostly to expansion of urban MCH services accompanied by a larger number of births in public sector hospitals in urban communities. MMR declined from 700 per 100,000 live births in 1947 to 396 in 1956 (same sources as in table 9).

The next phase (1957–75) was associated with the rapid establishment of an extensive network of rural health services as well as efforts to mobilize rural communities and encourage the use of services. Skilled attendance at childbirth in the homes of rural women expanded at a remarkable pace, and childbirth in public sector hospitals continued to rise. At the same time, MMR declined from 282 in 1957 to 83 in 1975.

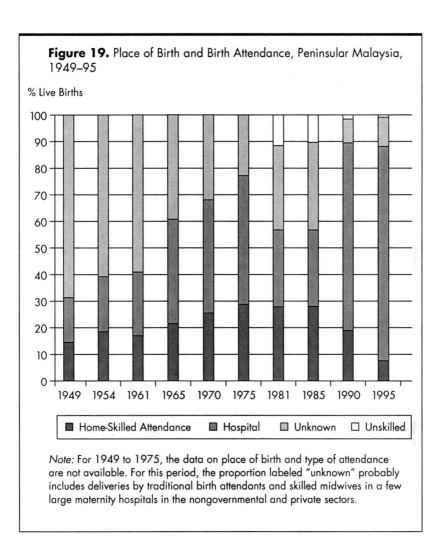

Figure 19. Place of Birth and Birth Attendance, Peninsular Malaysia, 1949–95

% Live Births

Home-Skilled Attendance   Hospital   Unknown   Unskilled

Note: For 1949 to 1975, the data on place of birth and type of attendance are not available. For this period, the proportion labeled "unknown" probably includes deliveries by traditional birth attendants and skilled midwives in a few large maternity hospitals in the nongovernmental and private sectors.

The third phase (1976–89) brought further growth in skilled attendance coverage (from about 70 percent to about 90 percent), including a strong shift among women in rural areas to giving birth in public sector hospitals and a marked upsurge in the number of women with complications of pregnancy being admitted to hospitals. This phase was marked by an emphasis on improved clinical and organizational management (Raj Karim, Ravindran, and Mahani

Table 9. Overview of Health Service Capacity and Skilled Attendance during Childbirth, Peninsular Malaysia, 1949–95

YEAR	MMR	BIRTHS WITH SKILLED ATTENDANCE (%)	LIVE BIRTHS PER MIDWIFE	LIVE BIRTHS PER NURSE+MIDWIFE	POPULATION PER DOCTOR	RATIO OF MIDWIVES AND NURSES TO 100 GOVERNMENT DOCTORS	HOSPITAL BEDS PER 1,000 POPULATION
1949	534	32	—	—	—	—	—
1952	520	—	461	138	8,727	648	2.46
1954	476	39	479	—	—	n.a.	n.a.
1956	396	—	506	—	—	599	—
1958	277	—	439	—	7,040	—	—
1960	242	—	316	125	6,857	578	2.04
1961	200	41	320	118	6,509	606	—
1965	204	61	197	81	5,654	648	—
1970	148	67	149	62	3,859	598	—
1975	83	76	122	52	4,084	472	1.76
1980	63	—	101	34	3,252	541	1.71
1985	37	—	108	32	2,859	615	1.6
1990	20	89	102	29	2,294	494	1.49
1995	21	87	115	29	1,960	374	1.41

— Not available.

MMR = Maternal mortality ratio.

Note: "Nurses" includes those with and without midwifery training. "Midwives" includes midwives and community nurse–midwives.

Sources: Federation of Malaya various years; City Council of George Town, 1946–69; Kuala Lumpur City Council various years; Malaysia, Ministry of Health various years; Malaysia Department of Statistics, 1991 and 2001.

2000). MMR declined from 78 per 100,000 live births in 1976 to 20 per 100,000 live births in 1989. The most recent phase began around 1990; it has been associated with an ever-increasing demand for childbirth in hospitals and a growth in the number of births in private hospitals.

Key Policies and Program Interventions

Key policies and program interventions supportive of maternal health were implemented in progressive incremental steps in the health sector and in related sectors to address priority problems and issues during successive phases of development. The focus of those policies and programs is illustrated in figure 20. During the initial phase, midwifery was professionalized through legislation and certification that was based on stringent training criteria. Birth and death registration was established, and models for maternal health care delivery were developed in urban areas. By the end of this period, maternal health was improving in urban communities, but rural areas had poor access to health services.

The next phase focused on improving access for rural communities through removal of geographic, financial, and cultural barriers to maternal health care and community mobilization. By the end of this phase, an extensive rural health service network had been established, but not all women who needed care used the services in a timely manner. The focus shifted to improving the quality of care, including referrals, and strengthening community involvement so as to ensure that available health services were utilized appropriately. Toward the end of this phase, demand for childbirth in hospitals increased, leading to overcrowding of tertiary care institutions. The focus has now expanded to coping with demand while maintaining quality.

The next two sections describe the societal environment that facilitated and sustained policies and programs for improving maternal health and the implementation of health program interventions to address critical problems during the different phases of health systems development.

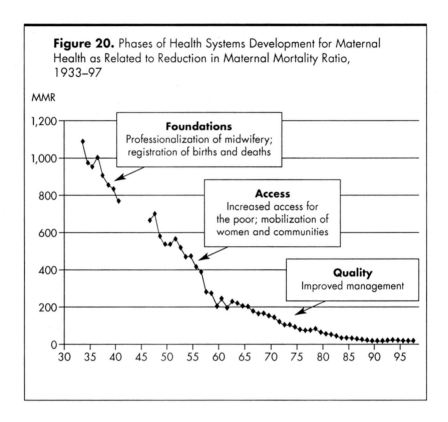

Figure 20. Phases of Health Systems Development for Maternal Health as Related to Reduction in Maternal Mortality Ratio, 1933–97

Forty Years of Supportive Policies and Social Programs (1957–97)

Several policies and social programs provided a supportive environment for maternal health throughout the second half of the 20th century. National policies recognized that health was important, and the government steadily invested in public health programs. Since Independence, political commitment to the reduction of urban–rural differences in development and to the reduction of social and economic imbalances has remained high. Relevant policies and programs that have been implemented in sequential, though overlapping, phases have included integrated rural development, empowerment and education of women, poverty reduction, urban development, and quality improvement (Government of Malaysia various years).

A high level of political commitment to improving MCH has been sustained for more than 60 years. Public investments in health, specifically in maternal health, have been modest but effective. Fertility has fallen, although the decline has been limited. Synergistic packages of effectively implemented policies and programs have addressed poverty and women's empowerment and improved physical access in rural and remote communities, thereby providing good access to mostly free health care, including maternity-related services and primary education. The next sections elaborate on each of these issues.

Rural Development. The government embarked on an integrated process of rural development that aimed to increase agricultural capacity and employment and involved improvements in transportation, energy supply, and the social sector. As a result, the rural population gained access to basic services, including health, education, roads, sanitation, and water supply. Local demand for rural development, which was channeled through elected political representatives, reinforced pressure on the government to provide these basic services (Government of Malaysia various years; Government of Malaysia 1991; Rahmah 1998).

Empowerment of Women. Women were given voting rights with Independence, and female education was promoted. Rural development activities included adult literacy classes, which served as vehicles to involve rural women and raise awareness about healthy behavior and covered topics including nutrition, childbirth and child care, and sanitation. In later years, the classes were converted to early childhood education programs (Rohana 1986). Efforts to improve women's status involved an even greater effort to promote girl's education, and female literacy increased from 49 percent in 1970 to 67 percent in 1990, narrowing the male–female literacy ratio from 1.45:1 to 1.21:1.

Poverty Reduction. Political pressures resulted in a strong emphasis on policies and programs to correct the imbalance between the ethnic groups. Poverty levels declined dramatically: the proportion of households in poverty dropped from 49 percent in 1970 to 8 percent in 1999 (12 percent rural and 3 percent urban). Sustained efforts were made to reduce gaps between the top and bottom 20 percent of the population, and the Gini coefficient[2] decreased from 0.513 in 1970 to 0.464 in 1995 (Fadil 1997; Government of Malaysia 2000).

Urbanization and Access. From 1981 to 1990 the country also experienced some socioeconomic changes that probably contributed to further growth in the utilization of maternity-related services. Following a recession in the early 1980s, manufacturing became the major source of economic growth. This shift was accompanied by large internal migration that changed the rural–urban distribution of the population (Government of Malaysia various years). Improved roads also facilitated transportation and access to health facilities in urban centers. By 1997, 90 percent of households had a safe water supply. In 1990, about 71 percent of the poor people in Peninsular Malaysia were located within 5 kilometers of rural clinics, where they could obtain free health care (Public Health Institute 1997).

Quality Improvement. Quality improvement became a national movement in the 1980s. The policy was implemented through a range of activities, beginning with all public sector activities that provided "counter services" to the public, such as mail, health, road transportation, and immigration. Hospitals and health centers across the country figured prominently as success stories of government services that had improved their image and provided more sensitive and caring services (Abu Bakar and Jegathesan 2000).

International Support. Some international agencies influenced health policy development during this period, including the World Health Organization (WHO), which provided a full-time consultant who had a critical role in designing MCH services, and the U.N. Fund for Population Activities. The World Bank, Asia Development Bank, and the United Nations Children's Fund provided critical analyses and or influenced the use of their loans (Abdul Khalid Sahan, informant interview).

Health Status. Between 1957 and 1975, life expectancy increased from 56 to 64 years for males and from 58 to 69 for females. A nationwide malaria eradication program was implemented, and malaria incidence declined to 412 cases per 100,000 population.

Fertility Reduction. Fertility was reduced from a total fertility rate (TFR)[3] of 6.7 in 1957 to 3.2 in 1999. This decline is significant but smaller than the dramatic decline in maternal mortality over the same period. The sharpest decline occurred during the 20-year period between 1960 and 1980, when TFR fell from 6.0 to 3.9. Over the same period, MMR fell from 282 to 63 maternal deaths per 100,000 live births. Subsequently, a pronatalistic policy was adopted, and since 1984 the proportion of women using contraception has remained between 50 and 55 percent. TFR has remained at 3.3 to 3.4, whereas maternal mortality and other health indicators, such as infant mortality, have declined steadily (Malaysia, Ministry of National Unity and Social Development 1999).

Two noteworthy features of fertility decline could be related to maternal mortality. First, differences in fertility between ethnic groups became substantial after the late 1970s: ethnic Malays experienced a slow decline compared with the other ethnic groups (table 10). Second, the fall in fertility has been greater for women younger than age 20 and older than age 40. In the two decades from 1960 to

Table 10. Total Fertility Rates, by Ethnic Group, Peninsular Malaysia, 1957–97

	TFR				
YEAR	MALAYS	CHINESE	INDIANS	OTHERS[a]	PENINSULAR MALAYSIA
1957	6.1	7.4	8.0	5.0	6.7
1960	5.7	6.3	7.3	5.3	6.0
1965	5.5	5.6	6.7	4.4	5.6
1970	5.1	4.6	4.8	4.3	4.9
1975	4.6	3.6	3.9	2.9	4.2
1980	4.5	3.1	3.4	3.0	3.9
1985	4.8	2.7	2.9	3.5	3.9
1990	4.1	2.3	2.6	3.8	3.3
1995	4.0	2.5	2.7	2.5	3.3
1997	3.8	2.5	2.6	2.9	3.3

[a]The TFR for this group is not available for 1957; TFR for 1958 is shown instead.
Sources: Malaysia, Department of Statistics 1991 and various years.

1980, TFR dropped by 35 percent, but the fertility of women ages 15 to 19 fell by 69 percent, that of women ages 40 to 44 fell by 40 percent, and that of women ages 45 to 49 fell by 71 percent. Reductions in age-specific fertility among the main ethnic groups in these three age bands were achieved in a beneficial way from a maternal mortality perspective: the higher the age-specific fertility in each ethnic group in these ages, the greater the drop in the age-specific fertility for the particular ethnic group. However, it is appropriate to point out that although maternal death rates among women ages 40 to 49 are higher than for younger ages, the proportion of women in this age group who bear children is less than 10 percent of the total (Malaysia, Department of Statistics 1991; Malaysia, Department of Statistics various years). Consequently, the observed reduction in fertility in the oldest age bracket could have had only a relatively small impact on aggregate MMR.

Public Expenditures on Health

The reduction in maternal mortality and other health improvements was achieved with a relatively modest outlay of public funds. Between 1946 and 1997, Malaysia spent about 1.4 to 1.8 percent of its gross domestic product (GDP) building and operating its comprehensive and mostly free publicly funded health services, a notable achievement. Briefly, the pattern of public expenditures on health services reflects different stages of health development and concern. Before Independence, both capital and operating expenditures were relatively low—less than 1 percent of GDP—because of the emphasis on providing disease-control and hospital services to the better-off population living in urban areas.

Three major periods are discernable (table 11). The first was during the 10 years prior to Independence (1946–55), when capital investment in new health facilities was relatively low. Increases in operating expenses can be attributed to a great extent to the filling of professional posts that had been depleted during World War II. The number of admissions to public hospitals per head of population did not increase, and the number of hospital beds per 1,000 population actually decreased over the period.

Table 11. Expenditures on Public Health, Malaysia, 1946–95

	EXPENDITURES (% OF GDP)		
PERIOD	OPERATING	CAPITAL	ALL
1946–50	0.69	0.01	0.70
1951–55	0.91	0.04	0.95
1956–60	1.40	0.14	1.54
1961–65	1.42	0.29	1.71
1966–70	—	0.28	—
1971–75	1.59	0.20	1.79
1976–80	1.49	0.14	1.63
1981–85	1.37	0.21	1.59
1986–90	1.31	0.19	1.51
1991–95	1.18	0.27	1.44

— Not available.
GDP = Gross domestic product.
Sources: Authors' compilation of data from various sources.

The second period covers the next 20 years, 1956–75. With Independence came a sevenfold upsurge in public sector capital expenditures for health services, reflecting rapid expansion in capacity and use of rural health services as well as hospitals. About 1,280 new midwife clinics[4] were built, which were backed by some 256 small health subcenters and 65 main health centers.[5] General and district hospital capacity rose by about 5,100 beds (an increase of 38 percent), and admissions increased from 44 per 1,000 population in 1960 to 59 per 1,000 population in 1975 (an increase of 34 percent; Malaysia, Ministry of Health various years). Staff increased significantly; for example, in the 2-year period from 1973–75 alone, the number of nursing staff and midwives employed increased by 27 percent. Nevertheless, operating expenditures increased at a slower pace than investment and reached their peak of 1.6 percent of GDP during 1971–75. Even at the height of capacity building and operating expenses, Malaysia's public sector expenditures on health services reached only 1.8 percent of GDP.

The third period was from 1976–95. The extensive rural health system had been established, and total public sector expenditures on health services declined to an average of 1.4 percent of GDP from 1991–95. Capital expenditures initially declined in relation to GDP, but investments in hospitals kept public capital expenditures on health services at around 0.2 percent of GDP. Subsequent years saw capital expenditures reach high levels (0.27 percent of GDP) as a result of increasing investments in hospitals, while a large decline occurred in the proportion spent on rural health services. Investment in hospitals mostly involved updating existing facilities, and inpatient capacity rose by fewer than 1,000 beds in Peninsular Malaysia. In fact, the higher rate of population growth led to an actual reduction in the number of public hospital beds for acute care from 1.8 per 1,000 population in 1975 to 1.2 per 1,000 population in 1995. The rate of use of acute inpatient services[6] remained about the same, at 50 admissions per 1,000 population. Despite the decline in the number of public hospital beds, the supply of beds continued to be well above demand. In 1995, on average, only about 60 percent of public hospital beds were occupied.

The operating expenditures of health services in the public sector gradually declined from their peak in 1971–75 (1.6 percent of GDP) to a low of 1.2 percent of GDP in 1991–95. This reduction in operating expenditures in relation to GDP kept total public sector health care expenditures at its lowest 5-year average (1.4 percent of GDP) since Independence. This phenomenon can be partly attributed to the lower personnel salary rates in relation to per capita GDP over time.

This study analyzes expenditures related to maternal health care against this dynamic background of public expenditures on the whole range of health services.

Public Expenditures on Maternal Health

One cannot estimate and analyze capital expenditures for maternal health care until the mid-1960s or estimate and analyze operating expenditures until the 1970s. By this time, rural health services had been established and substantial coverage had been achieved.

In the 25-year period from 1971–95, Malaysia spent an average of only 0.38 percent of GDP on the provision of maternal health care[7] (table 12). That spending included capital expenditures on facilities for a comprehensive and far-reaching network of community- and hospital-based services as well as operating expenses. The country

Table 12. Estimated Public Sector Expenditures on Maternal Health Care, Malaysia, 1971–95

TYPE OF EXPENDITURE	% GDP
Operating (total)	0.32
MCH	0.19
Hospital deliveries and complications	0.13
Capital (total)	0.06
MCH	0.04
Hospital deliveries and complications	0.02
All (total)	0.38
MCH	0.23
Hospital deliveries and complications	0.15

MCH = Maternal and child health.
Sources: Authors' compilation of data from various sources.

regards the relatively small proportion of GDP spent on maternal health care as eminently affordable.

Operating expenditures for maternal health care accounted for an average of 0.32 percent of GDP, which was less than one-fifth (18 percent) of the public expenditures on operating health services. Operating expenditures for maternal health care in hospitals were only 0.13 percent of GDP. On average, in the 25-year period 1971–95, total capital expenditures on maternal health care amounted to a humble 0.06 percent of GDP.

Affordability to Households

Improving health care services in rural areas was part of the Malaysian government's strategy to alleviate poverty. In accordance with that policy, antenatal care and home deliveries by government midwives and nurses were free. The free nature of the government service actually caused acceptability problems because it threatened the livelihood of traditional birth attendants (TBAs) in the villages. Consequently, the government deliberately made an effort to include TBAs in the strategy and provided a subsidy for their own work (Abdul Khalid Sahan, informant interview). Fees for hospital services depended on the level of hospital accommodation and the income of the person admitted. Admission to a third-class hospital was free for people with low incomes. However, fees even for the nonpoor were minimal and often not pursued. Data for 1976–77 show that collected fees represented the equivalent of only about 4 percent of the operating expenditures of hospitals (Malaysia, Ministry of Health various years).

A World Bank study in the 1970s showed that "more than two-thirds of hospital inpatients paid no fees; the same was true of more than three-quarters of outpatient treatment at all facilities. Regression analysis, with the various procedures as dependent variables, rejected income as an explanatory variable" (Young, Bussink, and Hasan 1980, p. 139). Another, more recent, World Bank study arrived at similar findings (Hammer, Nabi, and Cerone 1995). However, the findings of the later study have another facet to them: they show that the use of free health services provided by the government accounted for the equivalent of almost one-fifth of the income of the poorer households in Malaysia (Hammer, Nabi, and Cerone 1995).

Health Policy and Program Implementation: The Foundations (1933–57)

Policies and programs introduced by British colonial administrators prior to World War II were the foundation on which the future Malaysian health system developed. Thus, modern medicine as it was practiced in Britain in the first half of the 20th century influenced health services development in colonial Malaya. Critical to maternal health were the professionalization of midwifery, birth and death registration systems, establishment of models of MCH services that proved to be popular and encouraged skilled care during childbirth, and official recognition of MCH as a national priority. The measures were put in place when MMR was reportedly higher than 700 deaths per 100,000 live births, although it is believed that MMR was actually much higher because deaths were grossly underreported and health services were confined largely to urban areas.

Professionalization of Midwifery. Midwifery was professionalized through legislation governing the practice of midwifery, midwifery training, certification of midwives, and close supervision of midwives by nurse–midwives and nursing sisters. Midwifery legislation was enacted in different years during the first half of the 20th century in the various states of Malaya, consolidated in 1955, and updated several times during the subsequent decades (Malaya 1955, and Malaysia 1968, 1971, 1972, 1985, 1990). The midwifery curriculum, introduced during the colonial era (Manderson 1996), later proved to be feasible for large-scale replication. Although programs and services before Independence were limited to urban areas, their pattern provided the model for future development.

Midwives were registered under the Midwives Act and employed in the public sector. They had 18 months of rigorous clinical training in hospitals and home settings, and they visited the homes of pregnant women and of women who had reported a birth to the local registrar. They urged clinic attendance and provided free, clinic-based antenatal care as well as 10 days of postnatal care in clients' homes. They also managed childbirth in the homes of women who were reluctant to go to the hospital. In hospitals, the midwives conducted all normal deliveries.

Certified nurse–midwives closely supervised government midwives. Nurse–midwives were certified graduates of a 3-year basic nursing program, followed by 12-month midwifery training (9 months in hospitals and 3 months in domiciliary settings). They were registered under the Nursing and the Midwifery Acts. Some nurse–midwives had an additional 1-year training in public health to become public health nurses (PHN). The nurse–midwives and PHNs conducted prenatal and child health clinics, including nutrition education; responded to calls for help from midwives during home deliveries; helped arrange transportation for emergencies; spearheaded efforts to bring health information to communities; and mobilized local leaders to appreciate and respond to dangers during pregnancy and childbirth (Chong 1971; Nursing Division 1988).

Birth and Maternal Death Registration and Monitoring. Births and deaths were reported at local police stations, which are the peripheral sources of data for the registrar general (RG). Government midwives obtained information on maternal deaths from the local police station, thereby creating the earliest linkage between the health and civil registration systems for monitoring maternal deaths in the community. The practice of investigating maternal deaths was introduced during the colonial administration, albeit in an ad hoc manner and mostly in hospitals. This system gradually evolved into a full-fledged modern system of confidential inquiry into maternal deaths.

Maternal and Child Health Clinics and Home Visits. Prior to World War II, in response to concerns about high infant mortality, colonial authorities established a limited number of infant welfare clinics (later known as MCH clinics) in urban centers. The clinics had female staff provide child health care as well as antenatal and postnatal care for pregnant women. Staff encouraged childbirth in government hospitals that had beds set aside for maternity. During that era, the ethnic Chinese community also established private, not-for-profit maternity hospitals in the major townships; they were largely intended to serve the increasing number of female labor immigrants who lived in overcrowded housing with no facilities for childbirth at home. By the 1930s, recognizing the need to have midwives who were culturally acceptable to the community, authorities in some of the states made early efforts to encourage local Malay girls to train as midwives and be employed by local public sector authorities. Their clients were mainly Malays in periurban areas. Although little expenditure data are available, reports indicate that resource limitations, such as insufficient budget, lack of trained personnel, lack of rural infrastructure, and administrators' perceptions about cultural barriers among rural ethnic Malays limited the programs to urban areas. Some states, however, introduced measures in rural areas to increase community awareness of basic health and hygiene issues through such means as home science in girls' school curriculum and educating TBAs in clean delivery practices (Manderson 1996, Phua 1987).

During 1946–60, MCH clinics and maternity wards proved to be popular in urban and periurban areas; attendance at the clinics and home visits by midwives increased tenfold. Skilled attendance at delivery rose from 30 percent to about 40 percent, and almost all such childbirth for which records exist occurred in government hospitals and a couple of private Chinese maternity hospitals. MMR declined from more than 700 per 100,000 live births in 1947 to 396 in 1956. The fall in MMR among ethnic Chinese, who made up about 35 percent of the population, was most impressive. Chinese were more urban than the other ethnic groups, and the large-scale resettlement of rural ethnic Chinese into new villages during the late 1950s provided them easy access to MCH clinics and hospitals. By the end of this phase, MMR of ethnic Chinese was 140, compared with 200 and 400, respectively, among the predominantly rural ethnic Indians and Malays, who made up approximately 10 percent and 50 percent of the population

Effects of Major Health Problems on the Progress in Maternal Health. During the late 1940s and 1950s, the highest priority was given to overcoming the malnutrition that had become serious during the war years, to improving child survival and maternal health, and controlling communicable diseases. Malaria control measures, mostly environmental in nature, were reestablished in urban areas and for the labor force on the rubber estates. However, malaria remained a major problem for 60 percent of the population in rural areas. Although no national data exist prior to the 1960s, it is estimated that in the late 1950s and early 1960s, malaria incidence was about 2,300 cases per 100,000 population (Sandosham 1965).

Maternal and Child Health as National Priorities. In 1948, following the lead provided by WHO, the government identified maternal health as a top national priority and focused on expanding MCH services to the rural population. (Noordin 1978). A World Bank mission in 1955 noted that "the medical and health services of the Federation have been eminently effective in achieving a relatively high level of health....The maternity and child welfare field is one of the most rapidly growing areas of the Medical Department activity" (IBRD 1955).

Improving Access and Service Utilization by the Rural Poor (1957–75)

In the mid-1950s, female literacy was only 17 percent, and more than 60 percent of the population lived in rural areas, where health facilities were scarce. Nationwide, about one MCH clinic existed for every annual 1,000 live births, and about 480 live births occurred per midwife annually. The rural health service program was designed to improve access to a basic package of community-based services, including care during pregnancy, childbirth, and the postnatal period; child health and nutrition; communicable disease control; safe water and sanitation; and medical care for common illnesses. The initial thrust was on construction of clinic facilities and residential accommodations for staff, provision of transportation, and building of training facilities. This initial drive was soon complemented by the expansion of public hospital services: general and district hospital capacity rose by some 5,100 beds, or 38 percent (Malaysia, Ministry of Health, various years). About 12 percent of all beds were maternity beds. MCH clinic services and home visits were free for the clients, and childbirth in institutions was practically free except for those who chose to use first-class wards. The rapid expansion of the infrastructure managed to increase health service availability and access despite the high population growth (table 9). By 1977, surveys showed that more than 85 percent of the rural population lived within 3 miles of a static health facility, and mobile health teams served those who lived beyond that range (Noordin 1978). Today, the network of rural health services continues to be vital in providing access to services to families in rural areas.

Staffing Patterns. Four categories of staff contributed to various degrees to maternity services: government midwives and their supervisors; nurse–midwives; medical officers, who did not have postgraduate training in obstetrics; and specialist obstetricians. The midwives became the backbone of maternity services and provided the bulk of first-contact maternity services[8] in clinics, outreach home visits, and hospital labor rooms and maternity wards. To meet the needs of the rapidly growing population and expanding rural health services, the licensing of midwives and nurses doubled in 1971 and further increased during the subsequent 10 years. Access to skilled midwives improved as the ratio of government midwives to live births fell from more than 1:300 in 1960 to about 1:120 in 1975. Trained midwives became one of the cornerstones in the development of the highly successful rural health services of modern Malaysia. After the 1978 Alma Ata Declaration, the responsibilities of midwives were expanded to those of a community nurse, and the range of their activities widened to include child health (immunization and growth monitoring) and basic treatment of a few common conditions. However, their midwifery functions did not diminish. The prestige they had gained in the community as midwives enabled them to rapidly grow into their expanded role (Malaysia, Ministry of Health 1991, 1992).

Nurse–midwives were key figures. In hospitals, they managed the labor ward and supervised trained midwives, who managed normal deliveries, to ensure compliance with clinical management protocols. They dealt with the emergencies that arose during childbirth in hospitals that had no doctors with training in obstetrics (box 2). In the rural health services, supervisory nurses were nurse–midwives or PHNs. Not only did they provide hands-on support for midwives when complications arose during childbirth, but they also were effective and respected communicators at the village level. Nurse–midwives intensified community awareness of the dangers during pregnancy and childbirth and facilitated emergency transportation planning for remote communities.

Doctors did not provide first-contact maternity care, but they were the first line of referral for nurse–midwives. Doctors who did not have postgraduate training in obstetrics provided backup for nurse–midwives in recognizing complications in pregnancy and childbirth, provided emergency resuscitation, and performed a limited number of nonsurgical interventions. The number of doctors in the public sector was limited, however, and they served mostly in larger cities. About 600 nurses and midwives existed for every 100 doctors. Few private sector doctors provided maternity care.

In 1960, only five obstetricians were in the public sector (56,000 live births per obstetrician). By 1974, their number had increased to 25 (12,400 live births per obstetrician). During the 1960s, general surgeons provided emergency obstetric care in hospitals that had no obstetrician. In 1972, there were 2.1 acute hospital beds per 1,000 population. Although all 58 public sector hospitals had maternity wards, only 21 had maternity units with obstetricians.

Midwifery in Hospitals. In all hospitals, demand for maternity beds was high, and occupancy rates reached 100 percent in urban hospitals. Women who had an uncomplicated childbirth went home within 12 hours. Women who experienced complications during childbirth at home were brought to the nearest hospital, which could be a small hospital with no obstetrician. All such hospitals maintained a stock of emergency blood that was given prior to transport to the nearest large hospital. The shortage of doctors was a major problem that was aggravated by the continuing outflow of doctors, who were attracted by higher incomes and social amenities in urban areas, from the public to the private sector. Hospitals that had no doctors with specialist qualifications were underutilized because they provided only basic laboratory investigations and did not perform surgical interventions.

Partnership with Traditional Birth Attendants

In 1960 unskilled birth attendants handled about 60 percent of births; most of them were TBAs in rural areas. The need to overcome cultural barriers to the use of modern midwifery was recognized, and a partnership mode developed between government midwives and the local TBAs who had been the mainstay of village obstetrics. TBA practices were studied, documented, and classified into three categories: (a) harmful, and to be discouraged, (b) beneficial and to be encouraged, and (c) neutral, to be left undisturbed. It also became apparent that the introduction of free midwifery services by government midwives would generate hostility from the TBAs. Consequently, government staff was encouraged to work in partnership with TBAs. The latter were persuaded to provide harmless and much valued childbirth-

Box 1. Midwives and Nurse–Midwives in the 1960s and 1970s

"Those were the heady days of nation building. I worked in one of the most remote districts in Peninsular Malaysia and look back on those days with pride and affection. It was a privilege to have served our people and brought progress to our rural sisters. We nurses worked as a team and had a strong sense of ownership in the service that we provided. There were few doctors in the rural areas. It was up to us midwives and nurses. Midwives followed rigid clinical protocols that spelt the 'Do's and Don'ts' and were the backbone of their training. Each of us was held accountable. Everyone regarded a maternal death as a major tragic event."

Ajima Hassan, public health nurse–midwife

"Undaunted by physical hardships and lack of social amenities, nurses are found in the most remote parts of our country. This grit, this courage. All of you as a group should be proud of it. It is my earnest hope that this commitment shall continue to be a part of your profession and to burn as an eternal flame."

Abdul Khalid Sahan, former director general of health,
Malaysia, addressing nurses in 1984

"In the 1970s, I was in charge of a district hospital when the local leaders of a rural Malay community came to me in protest saying, "How can this young Chinese midwife help our women in childbirth? She does not know our customs

related services, such as postnatal massage, while the government midwife dealt with the childbirth process. TBAs were registered in a separate section of the Midwives' Register. They were trained in the avoidance of harmful practices and given an allowance of RM10 for each delivery they conducted. They were also provided with a kit for

Box 1. (continued)

and is not even married." I told them how well trained she was, and persuaded them to give her a try. Within a few months, they were singing praises about her dedication and usefulness to their villages."

Abu Bakar Suleiman, medical officer,
and former director general, Health Malaysia

"In those days, government employment was attractive, salaries were relatively high, and there was job security. Rural girls did not have many alternative careers. Midwifery and nursing were highly regarded professions for the educated girl."

Abdul Khalid Sahan, former director general of health, Malaysia

"Maternal death monitoring began in the 1950s. The importance of maternal mortality was enhanced by the investigation of each death by senior officials at state level. The physical presence of senior officials impressed the local staff and the involvement of the local community and the TBA in the investigations and discussions on each maternal death highlighted its seriousness."

Abu Bakar Suleiman and Ajima Hassan

hygienic care during childbirth. Registered TBAs reported their cases every month to the government midwife and had their supplies renewed. This approach was successful, and home deliveries shifted rapidly from TBAs to government-trained midwives.

Unsafe Abortion. As in most countries where abortion is illegal, complications of unsafe abortion have contributed to maternal deaths in Malaysia. A large community survey in 1977 found that 11 percent of women of reproductive age had had one or more induced abortions

Box 2: Midwifery Practice in Small Hospitals in the 1960s and 1970s

"There was no obstetrician, and it was the nurse–midwives who managed the labor room and looked after all obstetric problems. They called me only for a few complications, such as manual removal of the placenta. They knew which complications would require surgical intervention, and sent those promptly to the General Hospital."

Prabha, medical officer in Kuala Kangsar district hospital in 1966

"In the 1960s and early 1970s nurse–midwives were not allowed to give intravenous (IV) transfusion. But I had to transfer a patient to hospital 40 miles away and did not want to take a dead patient. Therefore I requested and obtained permission to let me start the IV drip. In Kelantan and Terengganu, where distances to hospital were long and there were frequent delays in transporting patients, nurse–midwives were allowed to give IV drips."

Rebecca John, nurse–midwife in Pontian district hospital in 1968

"In many places, I was the only obstetrician without even a medical officer to assist me. I had to train the nurse–midwives to give IV fluids and blood transfusion. Nurse–midwives did episiotomy and suturing of first-degree tear. Medical officers with some training in obstetrics did manual removal of placenta in smaller hospitals. Those without any training referred all the cases to the general hospitals. Blood was available at the smaller hospitals for emergencies."

T. Ng Khoon Fong, obstetrician in Perak, Kedah, and Johor from the 1960s to the mid-1970s

(Pathmanathan 1977). Review of government hospital records suggests that underreporting of abortion-related deaths was a major problem (Ng and Sinnathuray 1975). As in other countries, the complications of unsafe abortion often may be found under other diagnoses, such as bleeding or severe infection. However, the country adopted the same focused and pragmatic approach as for dealing with maternal deaths in general. Thus, adequate postabortion care was developed early and combined with appropriate contraceptive counseling and provision. In recent decades safe, legal abortion has become available for certain indications (Ravindran and Matthews 1996).

Expenditures on Maternal Health Care While Improving Access. Data constraints limit estimates of operating expenditures for maternal health care to the period after 1971. By this time a large network of nurses and midwives was working in rural as well as in urban MCH services; the ratio was about 1 midwife per 122 live births compared with 1 per 463 live births in 1955. Total public sector capital and operating expenditures on maternal health care constituted about 0.32 percent of GDP during the 5-year period, 1971–75. Operating expenditures amounted to 0.26 percent, and capital expenditures to 0.06 percent of GDP.

From 1966 to 1975, capital expenditures on rural health facilities related to maternal health care were 0.04 percent to 0.05 percent of GDP and supported a 32 percent increase in midwife clinics and rural health facilities in general along with a significant increase in training facilities. Capital expenditures on facilities for maternal health care in public hospitals were significant but modest, at about 0.01 percent of GDP between 1971 and 1975 (table 13).

Utilization of these services was high. MCH operating expenditures amounted to 0.17 percent of GDP during 1971–75; urban MCH services accounted for only 3 percent of the total. Operating expenditures for maternal health care in public hospitals amounted to the equivalent of about half of the expenditures on community-based MCH services (0.09 percent of GDP).

Table 13. Trends in Expenditures for Maternal Health Care, Malaysia, 1946–95

TYPE OF EXPENDITURE	1946–65	1966–70	1971–75	% OF GDP 1976–80	1981–85	1986–90	1991–95
Operating (total)	—	—	0.26	0.31	0.33	0.34	0.32
MCH	—	—	0.17	0.22	0.21	0.20	0.18
Hospital deliveries and complications	—	—	0.09	0.09	0.12	0.14	0.14
Capital (total)	—	—	0.06	0.05	0.08	0.06	0.05
MCH	—	0.04	0.05	0.04	0.06	0.04	0.02
Hospital deliveries and complications	—	—	0.01	0.01	0.02	0.02	0.03
All (total)	—	—	0.32	0.36	0.41	0.40	0.37
MCH	—	—	0.22	0.26	0.27	0.24	0.20
Hospital deliveries and complications	—	—	0.10	0.10	0.14	0.16	0.17

— Not available.
GDP = Gross domestic product.
MCH = Maternal and child health.
Sources: Authors' compilation of data from various sources.

Improving Utilization Through Better Management (1976–89)

By 1976 significant changes in women's empowerment had occurred. Female literacy had increased from 17 percent in 1957 to 49
percent in 1970, and the female–male literacy ratio had improved
from to 0.32 in 1952 to 0.47 in 1961 (table 4). Contraceptive prevalence had increased to 35 percent in 1975 (Nor, Ann, and Chee
1977). A wide network of rural health services had been established.
The training of midwives increased, and the number of midwives
annually licensed doubled by 1971, and the ratio of government
midwives to live births had improved from more than 1:300 in 1960
to about 1:120. The main thrust of health systems development had
shifted to improving quality through better organizational and clinical management. Implementation features are summarized in the
next few sections. The aim was further improvement in health and
appropriate utilization of available services.

MMR continued its steep descent from 78 to 20 maternal deaths
per 100,000 live births during this phase. By 1990, MMR had
reached 25 for ethnic Malays, 15 for Indians, and 9 for Chinese (table
8). The use of skilled attendance during childbirth increased from
about 80 percent in 1975 to almost 90 percent in 1990. Home deliveries by government midwives climbed rapidly during the first 10
years of this phase to reach a peak in 1986 (figure 19). At that time,
about 75 percent of live births had skilled attendance, and 1 in 4
births with skilled attendance was a home delivery by a government
midwife. During the next 10 years a rapid shift occurred toward
childbirth in a hospital. Pregnancy complications managed in government hospitals increased rapidly from an average of 83 admissions
per 1,000 live births during the period 1971–75 to 330 admissions by
the period 1986–90 (figure 21).

Capacity Upgrading in the Health Sector. During this third phase, particularly in the early years, increasing attention was given in rural
health services to the upgrading of existing physical facilities and
retraining of rural midwives to become community nurses capable of
providing basic child health, nutrition, and medical care. Hospitals
were upgraded, and the clinical competence of nurses and midwives

Box 3. The Referral Chain

"It was the rural health service expansion and the government midwives and nurses in the rural health services that were the critical factors in MMR reduction during the 1960s and 1970s. Also, the vehicles placed in rural health centers and smaller hospitals were very important in timely transport of patients. Government midwives were good at early recognition of complications of pregnancy and labor, and midwives and nurse–midwives were very effective in persuading patients who had complications to come to hospital. When a complication was detected, they would bring the patient to the nearest health center, where government transport was available to bring the patient to hospital. Small hospitals that did not have facilities for surgical interventions did have a stock of emergency blood (group O), which nurses and doctors administered to emergency cases prior to transport to a larger hospital. In larger hospitals that had no obstetrician, the general surgeon would perform emergency caesarian sections."

A. Tharmaratnam, obstetrician in Melaka, Perak,
and Penang during the 1960s

"The setting up of rural health infrastructure nearer to the community facilitated antenatal care whereby early detection especially of anemia could be corrected. Referral of complicated cases to hospitals was a crucial factor in saving women's lives. Although there were no proper roads to the interior areas, patients used to be carried across paddy fields in Kedah and were transported by the waiting ambulance to the hospital. Availability of transport and blood in the hospital was also important."

S. Maheswaran, obstetrician in Kedah, Negeri Sembilan, and
Perak in the 1960s and 1970s

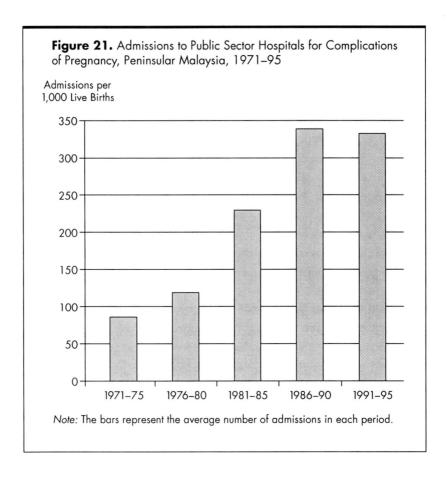

Figure 21. Admissions to Public Sector Hospitals for Complications of Pregnancy, Peninsular Malaysia, 1971–95

Admissions per
1,000 Live Births

Note: The bars represent the average number of admissions in each period.

in hospitals was raised through inservice training. Moreover, increasing numbers of doctors qualified in obstetrics and were placed in several smaller hospitals (Abu Bakar and Jegathesan 2000). The number of doctors employed in the public sector increased sharply, from 1,400 in 1975 to 4,000 in 1995, and the population per doctor (both public and private) declined from 4,084 to 1,960 (table 9).

Reducing Delays That Led to Maternal Death. During the 1980s and 1990s, the key feature of maternity-related services was improved patient management that had a phased focus on reducing delays that lead to maternal death. The initial emphasis during the early 1980s was on preventing delays in recognizing pregnancy complications and seeking help. During the second half of this period, the effort focused on delays in getting patients to the appropriate level of care and delays in providing appropriate clinical management at the institutional level. Thus, in the early years of the period, much attention was given to the community level, whereas in the later years, focus shifted to improving the coordination between rural health services and hospitals and to intrahospital measures.

Rural Health Service Management. Strengthening the management of MCH services began with the establishment of a small MCH unit in the MOH in 1971. During the 1980s management capacity was expanded through establishment of MCH management teams, including a medical officer trained in public health and senior nursing personnel, in every state. Monitoring of the MCH program was improved through standardization of reporting systems from rural health and hospital services. Regular performance reviews were undertaken to monitor progress in providing skilled attendance and antenatal and postnatal coverage. Districts and subdistricts that had below-average performance were subject to intensified management attention (Malaysia, Ministry of Health 1992). By this time, maternal death investigations had been systematized with standard formats and procedures that mandated involvement of supervisory nursing and medical personnel from the hospitals and rural health as well as community leaders. Subsequently, the system evolved into a full-fledged system of confidential inquiry into maternal deaths, with review of the compiled findings of all investigations. In 1991, a national committee was established to conduct this assessment (see below); it analyzed the collated findings of all inquiries on an annual basis.

A manual of procedures and clinical protocols for rural midwives was produced in 1988. The intensive inservice training of midwives and nurses in the rural health services included clinical as well as community mobilization aspects (Public Health Institute 1985, 1987). In response to international initiatives on the "Risk Approach," a study was undertaken in 1979 that resulted in the implementation in 1983 of a color-coding scheme intended to facilitate the referral of pregnant women by rural staff to appropriate levels of the health care system. Inservice management training courses used team problem-solving approaches to overcome communication and attitudinal barriers between hospital and rural health staff. They also built capacity to resolve local problems at that level (Public Health Institute 1983b). Although isolated evaluative studies of some of these initiatives (such as the Risk Approach) have not been able to demonstrate any significant impact on referral of complications of pregnancy, the increase in admissions for pregnancy complications attests to the effectiveness of the package of interventions implemented in Malaysia.

Improved Hospital and Clinical Management. Hospital management was also addressed. In 1986 a quality assurance program was initiated in hospitals; it included the systematic monitoring of specific aspects of quality of care and continuous quality improvement efforts. For example, eclampsia was used as a sentinel-event, or "marker–tracer condition," indicator that merited detailed investigation of why it had not been prevented. This approach encouraged the hospital-based obstetrician to take responsibility for quality of care in the entire health district and promoted coordination with the rural health services (Abu Bakar and Jegathesan 2000). Management training in problem solving for hospital teams included clinicians, nurses, and managers. Substantial attention was given to pregnancy complications missed in busy hospital prenatal clinics, and review of routine management procedures was encouraged. Clinical procedures, such as the routine use of partograms (graphic presentation of evolution of labor), were upgraded.

Confidential Inquiry into Maternal Deaths. By 1980, rural health services had been well established, skilled attendance had reached 70 percent, government midwives were actively looking for possible maternal deaths in the villages, and the MOH was recording the causes of death. Deaths with known causes were about equal in number to those reported to the registrar. Postpartum hemorrhage had declined dramatically, and associated medical conditions were becoming an important cause of death.

By 1990, skilled attendance had reached almost 90 percent. The efforts of MOH field personnel resulted in the identification of twice as many maternal deaths as those reported to the RG, and skilled attendance had reached 90 percent. In 1991, for the first time, a full-scale confidential inquiry into maternal death reviewed and analyzed all investigation reports in the MOH and found that 81 percent were due to obstetric complications. The leading causes of death were postpartum hemorrhage, hypertensive disorders of pregnancy, and pulmonary embolism. Most women had died after childbirth. The maternal death rate was 41 per 100,000 hospital deliveries and 52 per 100,000 home deliveries. Substandard care was noted in 46 percent of deaths. The report served as the basis for several remedial measures. Examples of some intrahospital measures include a "red alert" system to provide timely and adequate response to emergencies; revised clinical management protocols (for example, stabilization of critically ill patients prior to transport); and improved referral and feedback between hospitals and health centers (Malaysia, Ministry of Health 1998). The findings of the inquiry were used to formulate and revise clinical procedures for public sector hospitals (Malaysia, Ministry of Health 1991, 1994, 1997).

Expenditures on Maternal Health Care. During this consolidation phase, estimated total public expenditures for maternal health care hovered below 0.41 percent of GDP when it reached its peak in 1981–85. Two compensatory factors contributed to the relative stability of the estimate: a fall in the proportion of expenditures on community-based MCH services from a peak of 70 percent of maternal health care operating expenses to about 57 percent, and an increase in hospital maternal health services to about 43 percent. An initial increase in operating expenses of community-based MCH services occurred during 1976–80, when home deliveries reached their peak, followed by a steady decline during the next three 5-year periods, when childbirth shifted to hospitals. The initial increase was also partly due to a large increase in public servant salaries. However, greater use of hospitals for childbirth and complications of pregnancy brought the maternal health care share of capital expenditures in hospitals to about 0.02 percent of GDP during 1981–90.

The increased use of hospitals for childbirth resulted in increased operating expenditures for maternal health services in hospitals, from 0.09 percent in 1976–80 to 0.14 percent of GDP in 1991–95 (figure 22). As expected, salaries and other personnel expenses constituted the largest proportion of the operating expenditures of MOH-funded services. Salaries constituted about 74 percent of the operating expenditures of MCH services in 1985 but fell considerably, to only 64 percent of the total in 1995. Similarly, personnel expenses made up about 66 percent of hospital operating expenditures in 1985. Capital investment in rural health services fell during this period, and capital expenditures on upgrading of hospitals increased (figure 23).

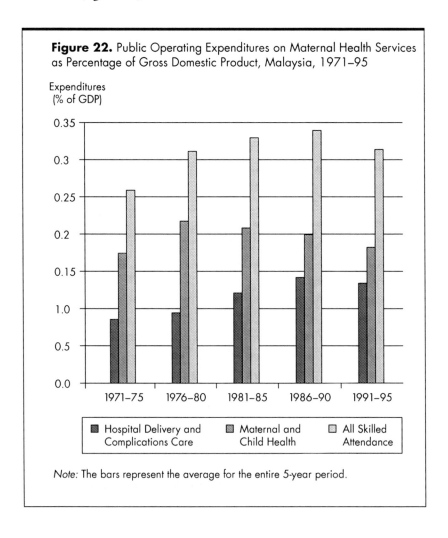

Figure 22. Public Operating Expenditures on Maternal Health Services as Percentage of Gross Domestic Product, Malaysia, 1971–95

Expenditures (% of GDP)

Legend:
- Hospital Delivery and Complications Care
- Maternal and Child Health
- All Skilled Attendance

Note: The bars represent the average for the entire 5-year period.

Coping with Increasing Demand (1990–97)

MMR fluctuated between 17 and 22 per 100,000 live births in the period after 1990. The reasons for this plateau are beyond the scope of this study; however, as stated in the section on confidential inquiry into maternal deaths, reporting of maternal deaths improved greatly after 1991. Therefore, estimates of actual levels of MMR during ear-

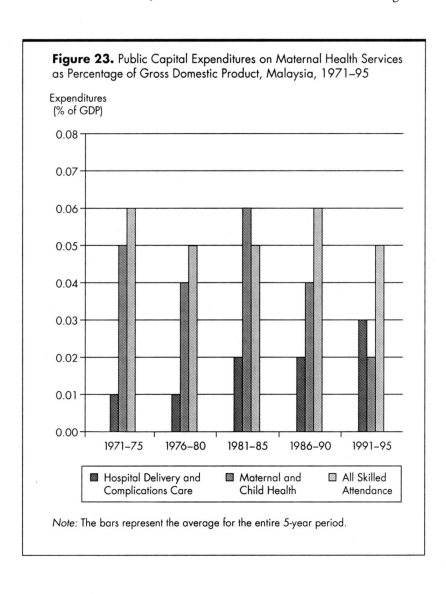

Figure 23. Public Capital Expenditures on Maternal Health Services as Percentage of Gross Domestic Product, Malaysia, 1971–95

Note: The bars represent the average for the entire 5-year period.

lier years are probably too low, although the MMR trends prior to the changed reporting process are probably fairly accurate. About 91 percent of live births had skilled attendance, and 87 percent were in hospitals. The proportion of childbirth in private hospitals increased during the 1980s to about 15 percent during the 1990s. The following sections describe some key features of this period.

Private Sector Growth. The late 1980s and the period from 1990 to 1996 were times of buoyant economic conditions that created additional demand for health care facilities. The number of private hospitals increased considerably, from 50 hospitals totaling 1,171 beds in 1980 to 203 hospitals totaling 7,471 beds in 1996. By 1996, the public sector provided 78 percent of the hospital bed capacity in Malaysia (including Sabah and Sarawak); private, for-profit hospitals supplied 17 percent of hospital beds; and not-for-profit hospitals provided 5 percent. A large proportion of the private hospitals were small (less than 20 beds), and most provided only maternity services.

Public Sector Expenditures on Skilled Attendance. By 1991–95, the proportion of total expenditures attributable to maternal health services was about 0.37 percent of GDP. This was a relatively small increase from expenditures in 1971–75 and was due entirely to the growth in expenditures related to maternal health services in public hospitals, which almost doubled in terms of percentage of GDP from 1971–75 to 1991–95. Over the same period, expenditures on community-based MCH services experienced a small reduction, from 0.22 percent of GDP in 1971–75 to 0.20 percent of GDP in 1991–95.

Conclusion

The Malaysian experience illustrates one model for reducing maternal mortality in a developing country using mainly public financing and provision of maternal health services. MMR reduction has been rapid and sustained. Health policies and programs evolved through successive phases of health systems development and were facilitated and supported by related policies in education, rural development, and poverty reduction. Success has been achieved with modest public expenditures on health and on maternal health care, and maternal health services have been largely free to clients who wanted them. An outstanding feature has been the success in making critical services accessible to the poor.

Notes

1. Skilled attendance refers to deliveries by clinically trained midwives and nurse–midwives, registered under the Midwives Act and by doctors. The actual services provided included antenatal as well as postnatal care.

2. The Gini coefficient is an indicator of income distribution; the higher the coefficient, the greater the inequality in income distribution. The lowering of the coefficient in Malaysia means that income inequality was reduced during that period.

3. TFR is the average number of children that a woman age 15 can expect to bear if she lives until at least age 50.

4. Midwife clinics had outpatient facilities for prenatal and child health care, but no maternity beds. Residential housing for the midwife was attached to each clinic.

5. Health centers and subcenters had outpatient facilities managed by doctors, nurses, and midwives and were the subdistrict facility responsible for outreach and public health services. They had no inpatient beds.

6. In Malaysia, acute hospitals provide skilled attendance of both complications of pregnancy and normal deliveries.

7. Maternal health services include both normal and complicated deliveries as well as episodes of care for complications of pregnancy

in public hospitals. Maternal health services also provide a whole range of maternal and child health services in community-based facilities during the antenatal and postnatal periods, including well-baby clinics, child immunization, and growth monitoring.

8.   The term "first contact" refers to the first contact between the pregnant woman and the maternal health service.

CHAPTER 3

Sri Lanka

Background: Sri Lanka Today

Sri Lanka is a densely populated island situated at the southern tip of
the Indian subcontinent. It has a multiethnic society of Sinhala (74
percent), who are predominantly Buddhists; Sri Lankan Tamils (12.6
percent) and Estate Tamils (5.6 percent), who are predominantly
Hindu; Moors and Malays (7 percent); and Burghers (0.8 percent)
(Sri Lanka Department of Census and Statistics 1996). The country
has a parliament and an executive president, who is assisted by a cab-
inet of ministers, all of whom are elected by the people. Classified as
a low-income developing country, Sri Lanka's human development
outcomes are on par with countries that have a much higher economic status (table 14).

Political and Social Context

Sri Lanka, formerly known as Ceylon, became an independent state
in 1948 and has remained a parliamentary democracy since then.
However, the country's history of more than 24 centuries has greatly
influenced its culture, educational development, and ethnic composition as well as its current political situation. Early incursions from
North India established the Sinhala kingdom in 543 B.C., which was
followed by almost 20 centuries of Sinhala Buddhist rule. The Sri

Table 14. Sri Lanka at a Glance

	AT INDEPENDENCE (1950)	MOST RECENT
Infant mortality per 1,000 live births	82	23[a]
Life expectancy (years) (males)	56	71[b]
Life expectancy (years) (females)	55	76[b]
Maternal mortality per 100,000 live births	555	15[c]
Total fertility rate	5.0	2.1
		(1995–2000)

	RECENT DATA
Female literacy rate (%)[d]	88
Female-to-male literacy ratio[d]	0.94
GNP per capita[e]	US$802
GNP per capita growth rate (%) (1998–99)	2.7
Households below the poverty line (%)[d]	35
Population (millions)[b]	18.5
Population growth rate per annum (%)[b]	1.0
Population in urban areas (%)[b]	23
Population less than age 20 (%)[f]	39
Population living within 1 hour of a health facility (%)	93
Population with access to safe drinking water (%)[e]	75
Population with access to sanitation (%)[e]	73
Skilled attendance at childbirth (%)[e]	97
Total health expenditures (% of gross domestic product)[b]	3.4

GNP = Gross national product.
[a]1997
[b]Hsiao 2000.
[c]1996
[d]1991 data.
[e]2000 estimates from DHS, excluding North and East.
[f]Estimates from the Demographic and Health Survey (DHS) 1993, excluding North and East.
Sources: UNDP (2000) and authors' compilation of data from various sources.

Lankan Tamil population originated with the repeated South Indian invasions during this period. Both Buddhist and Sri Lankan Tamil cultures place a high value on education. Buddhist culture and ideology have provided fertile ground for the welfare ideology that pervades the social sector of modern Sri Lanka and have supported the significant contribution women have made to social and human development in Sri Lanka (Gunatilleke 2000).

The colonial era began in 1505 and lasted almost 450 years; it consisted of successive rule by the Portuguese, Dutch, and finally, the British. This colonial heritage greatly influenced the modern-day political, legal, administrative, and health systems in Sri Lanka. The British era witnessed the development of the plantation industry: coffee at first, then tea and rubber. An important new element was added to the population through contracted south Indian labor that was brought to the island to work on the plantations. The subsequent development of the "Estate Tamils," as this group came to be known, was influenced by the fact that the employer, rather than the state, was mainly responsible for their welfare. Communication systems, an extensive network of roads and rail, Western medical services, and education in English were developed to support the plantation economy. A system of registration of vital events became operational in 1867 and drew attention to the common causes of death at that time. From as early as 1902, the Registrar General (RG) introduced a section in his annual reports highlighting the maternal mortality problem.

The development of specific services for mothers in Sri Lanka can be traced back to ancient and medieval times. A detailed town plan of Anuradhapura, the ancient capital of Sri Lanka, from the 4th century B.C., refers to a hospital and a "house of delivery" in this hospital complex (Fernando 1996). Kings built specialized hospitals, and the first maternity home was probably established between 522 and 524 A.D. (Uragoda 1987). It appears that Sri Lanka was among the pioneers in the provision of communal maternity homes. Medieval literature from the eighth and ninth centuries describes methods used in the treatment of abnormal parturition (Fernando 1996).

An important landmark in the socioeconomic development of Sri Lanka was the introduction of the elective principle as early as 1912, when "educated Ceylonese"[1] were given the vote; universal franchise was granted in 1931, long before national independence in 1948. It is said that the reason for women in Ceylon to be enfranchised was that "women's services would be of special value in coping with the high infant mortality rate in the island and with the need for better housing and improved midwifery and prenatal services" (Myrdal 1968, p. 344). The elected representatives were able to bring pressure on the executive for a larger allocation of resources for the provision of social services to the constituencies they represented. "Schools, rural hospitals, roads, and sub-post offices were the most common items in the list of demands" (Marga Institute 1984, p. 28). This effort led to an expanded program of construction of maternity homes, central dispensaries, rural hospitals, and cottage hospitals in areas that had been neglected. Direct taxation on income was introduced in 1932 and provided finances needed for the various welfare schemes (Meegama 1969). During this early phase, the government allocated substantial resources for expanding the state health system, including preventive and curative care. In 1928, 8 percent of government spending was for the health sector. Medical care was provided by the public sector free of charge, and a steady expansion of the system into rural areas—particularly in the 1930s and early 1940s—ensured access for the rural poor. The health sector focused attention on preventive care, particularly the control of major communicable diseases, although attention to maternal and child health (MCH) care increased during this period. Utilization of services was high, and it is believed that the use of health care services resulted in the rapid progress of social indicators during the subsequent post-independence era (Gunatilleke 2000).

The importance of education was acknowledged early and led to the rapid expansion of schools, especially in the first half of the 20th century, resulting in increasing levels of literacy (table 15). In 1945 education from school entry to university was declared free, stimulating unprecedented interest in education throughout the country.

Education spread widely and contributed to health improvement. Expansion of education enhanced the health consciousness of the people and increased utilization of health services that were provided free.

Study Approach

Sri Lanka's success in reducing maternal mortality has been widely discussed. Most studies have focused on specific aspects, such as trends in maternal mortality and causes of death (De Silva 2001),

Table 15. Trends in Adult Literacy, Sri Lanka, 1901–91

LITERACY	1901	1910	1921	1946	1953	1963	1971	1981	1991
Males (%)	42	47.2	56.4	70.1	75.9	79.3	85.6	91.1	90.2
Females (%)	8.5	12.5	21.2	43.8	53.6	63.2	70.9	83.2	83.1
Literacy ratio (Female:male)	0.20	0.26	0.38	0.62	0.71	0.80	0.83	0.91	0.92

Source: Authors' calculations based on data from the Department of Census and Statistics.

development of maternal health services (Fernando 1996), female literacy and empowerment (Gunatilleke 2000), malaria control (Abeyesundere 1976), and the relationship of maternity mortality ratio (MMR) and fertility (Seniveratne and Rajapaksa 2000; Dissanayake 1999). Some studies have reviewed maternal mortality within the context of intersectoral linkages to health (Gunatilleke 1984). Borghi (2000) compiled an extensive unpublished report exploring the relationship between health system development and reproductive health in Sri Lanka.

This study builds on previous work. It fills gaps in information, particularly with regard to use of skilled attendance and maternity care in institutions during different phases of health system development. It adds an in-depth dimension to the analysis of maternal health care development through information from key officials who had firsthand experience of the problems and the implementation strategies during critical earlier phases of development. This study compiles and analyzes public expenditures on maternal health care in conjunction with key features of health system development.

This chapter first examines temporal associations between trends in MMR and the use of skilled attendance and institutional childbirth, describes how the profile of maternal deaths changed as more women used skilled attendance and institutional facilities, and analyzes the relationship between fertility and MMR. Next, the chapter describes the development of maternal health services, namely, health infrastructure, human resource development, and management of MCH care. This material is followed by an analysis of the stepwise implementation of critical health policies and interventions to address key problems at different stages of health system development. Finally, the chapter provides an analysis of public expenditures on maternal health care and discusses the issue of affordability.

Maternal Mortality Data Availability and Quality

Intensive review of data sources used in previous studies revealed that some of the data required correction. The data used in this study are from the reports published by the RG. Completeness of birth and death registration data were studied for 1953, 1967, and 1980 and were found to be 89 percent, 95 percent, and 93 percent complete, respectively (Sri Lanka Ministry of Health 1993). Recently, however, the quality of data has deteriorated because of the civil war situation in the north and east, and studies have revealed a degree of underregistration of deaths.

A study carried out in 1994 and 1995 found 24 percent underreporting of maternal deaths in the Western Province (Bandhutilaka 1996). It has been suggested that the discrepancy between numbers reported at maternal death reviews and those reported by the registration system has increased in recent years (De Silva 2001). The increasing discrepancy may be a result of rising numbers of indirect causes of maternal death being reported through the field and hospital systems, following refresher education of health personnel on definition and reporting of maternal mortality.

Quality of Health Services Data

Health service data for the period 1900–57 are available from the reports of the director of Health Services (DHS); they have been available from the *Annual Health Bulletin* since 1980. Gaps in health service data exist for 1968–79, when health data were included in a brief manner in the general *Administration Reports;* the details given are inadequate for the present study. Unpublished data available from the Medical Statistics Unit have been used to supplement the above sources. Health service data do not include any information from the private sector. Institutional deliveries reported in health statistics are only those occurring in government institutions; here, too, the coverage may be incomplete because data from the northern and eastern provinces are not available for certain years.

The number of registered doctors, nurses, and midwives are available from the Sri Lanka Medical Council commencing from 1907, 1930, and 1949 respectively. Nurses with midwifery qualifications are entered in the register both as nurses and as midwives.

Information was also obtained from 15 key informants, including doctors, nurses, and midwives who had worked in health services at the district level and later became senior managers. The interviews covered issues such as perceptions regarding MCH services and obstetric practices from the late 1950s to the 1970s, the acceptance of midwives, the backup services available, and training during the early periods.

Expenditures and Affordability

The data used to estimate expenditures on skilled attendance are mainly from the annual reports of the DHS and are complemented by data from other published reports. For the period 1932–54, the annual administrative reports issued by the DHS provided comprehensive data on expenditures and admissions. The reports issued by the director general of Health Services (DGHS) provided aggregate recurrent expenditure figures for 1955–62. The 1960s and 1970s proved to be the most difficult period to examine; because detailed annual reports were not available for this period, health expenditure data were calculated using the ratios of health expenditures to gross domestic product (GDP) (1963–72) and government health expenditures to GDP (1973–79), as published by the Central Bank. For 1980–99, the *Annual Health Bulletin* proved to be a most valuable source of health expenditure and admissions data.

For each year under study, total expenditures were calculated on the basis of payroll data[2] and other expenditure data[3] available in the annual reports. Whenever possible, expenditures unrelated to maternal care[4] were excluded. Despite attempts to disaggregate payroll cost by staffing category [that is, midwives, public health midwives (PHMs), and so on], the lack of detailed data in all but the most recent years dictated that the expenditures on skilled attendance would be calculated by allocating total expenditures to maternity and nonmaternity functions by the ratio of maternity to nonmaternity admissions.

In assessing affordability to clients and households, information on policy was found in the *Annual Administration Report* and other published sources, which were complemented by information gathered in key informant interviews carried out in Colombo in June 2001.

Decline in Maternal Mortality Ratio

Sri Lanka's achievements in reducing the maternal mortality ratio have been one of the spectacular aspects of its success story in human development. Review of the time taken to reduce the MMR (maternal deaths per 100,000 live births) by 50 percent demonstrates an interesting pattern. It took 17 years (1930–47) for MMR to decline from more than 2,000 to about 1,000. In the next 3 years (1947–50), the MMR diminished a further 50 percent. Subsequent 50 percent reductions have been achieved during periods of 8 to 13 years (table 16).

Previous studies have discussed some of the temporal associations between MMR decline during various periods of time and other factors believed to have contributed to the decline. The steep decline in

Table 16. Time to Halve the Maternal Mortality Ratio, Sri Lanka, 1930–96

YEAR	MMR	INTERVAL (YEARS)
1930	2,136	n.a.
1947	1,056	17
1950	486	3
1963	245	13
1973	121	10
1981	58	8
1992	27	11
1996	24	4

n.a. Not applicable.
Source: Authors' compilation of data from various sources.

MMR that was observed from the 1930s to the early 1950s (see also figure 1, page 2) has been attributed largely to the all-out war against malaria (Abeyesundere 1976). DDT spraying commenced in 1945 and led to a rapid decline in malaria incidence within a few years. In addition to the highly successful malaria control program, it has also been suggested that control of hookworm infection and general improvements in sanitation contributed to the improvements in maternal health prior to 1950 (Wickramasuriya 1939). Moreover, it has been suggested that the rapid decline in MMR during the early 1950s could be attributed to the introduction of modern medical advances, such as antibiotics, through a health service network established in the pre-1950s era and having considerable reach in rural areas (Gunatilleke 2000).

Trends in Maternal Mortality Ratio and Female Death Rates

Figure 24 illustrates the relative change in the female death rate and MMR from 1950–96. In 1950, 8,933 female and 1,692 maternal deaths occurred among women ages 15 to 49; thus, the maternal deaths constituted 19 percent of female deaths. Forty-six years later, in 1996, the corresponding figures were 6,850, 81, and 1.2 percent. The relative changes in MMR and the female death rate were similar during the first 10-year period in that both showed a sharp decrease. Between 1960 and 1974 the decrease in the maternal death rate was much more pronounced; thereafter, the reduction in the relative change was similar. This trend indicates that factors affecting female deaths in general, such as improvements in the health infrastructure and general health status, had a greater impact during the first 10-year period. Specific factors may have acted to improve MMR thereafter. Records indicate that antenatal care was provided from as early as 1921 and that the number of mothers registered for antenatal care has shown a steady increase over time. In addition, food supplementation programs, in the form of milk-feeding centers for mothers and children, were established in the 1940s. Improvements in food supplies and in the general standard of living occurred

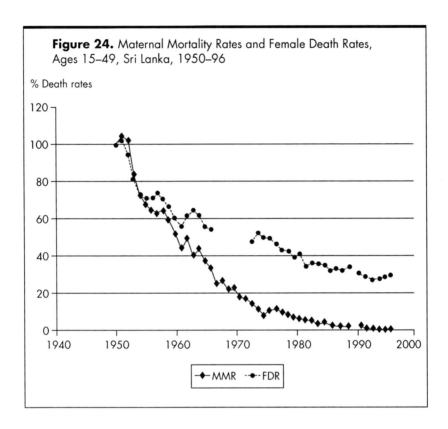

Figure 24. Maternal Mortality Rates and Female Death Rates, Ages 15–49, Sri Lanka, 1950–96

during the postwar period. The food rationing scheme introduced during the war was continued in the postwar period, ensuring a basket of goods at subsidized rates that was sufficient in quantity to ensure the minimum calorie requirement of an average family.

The food subsidy policies could not be maintained with the rapid expansion of the population and declining external earnings. Furthermore, the period 1973–75 brought circumstances that resulted in high food prices, the effects of which could not be ameliorated through the food ration scheme, resulting in an acute shortage of food. The adverse effects were reflected in the mortality and morbidity rates. The crude death rate and deaths among women of reproductive age increased during 1974–76. The infant mortality rate increased in 1974. A national nutrition survey in 1976 showed that 35 percent of children under 72 months were stunted and 6.6 percent were wasted (U.S. Centers for Disease Control and Prevention and others 1978). However, maternal mortality continued to decline.

Skilled Attendance during Childbirth

The trends in skilled attendance during childbirth and MMR are presented in table 17. Prior to 1940, less than 30 percent of live births had skilled attendance, and most such births took place in the client's home under the care of the public health midwife. During the 1940s, skilled attendance doubled. While skilled attendance in the client's home remained high, more women began to use institutional childbirth. A World Bank mission to Sri Lanka in 1952 noted the growing demand for institutional childbirth and the popularity of smaller rural institutions managed by midwives: "There are 113 maternity homes in the rural areas, sometimes located in out-of-the-way places. Practically everywhere one goes, be it a provincial, district, or rural hospital or maternity home, there are a large number

Table 17. Deliveries with Skilled Attendance and Maternal Mortality Ratio, 1939–95

YEAR	% ASSISTED DELIVERIES IN THE HOME	% DELIVERIES IN GOVERNMENT INSTITUTIONS	MMR
1939	19	8	1,824
1940	21	6	1,607
1945	27	22	1,694
1950	25	33	555
1955	25	41	405
1960	19	55	302
1965	15	62	239
1970	9	66	145
1975	—	67	102
1980	—	76	65
1985	—	75	51
1990	4	71	—
1995	2	87	24

— Not available.
Source: Authors' compilation of data from various sources.

of waiting maternity patients and like other hospital cases they are fed and treated free of charge" (IBRD 1952, p. 397). The mission noted that women "came to hospital days and even weeks before the actual time of childbirth" (IBRD 1952, p. 398), probably because of difficulties villagers encountered in transporting women in labor, especially at night.

The 1950s brought significant changes in the place of childbirth. Home deliveries began to decline as women increasingly sought delivery in institutions.[5] The role of the PHM in the community gradually changed from attending to births in the home to managing or assisting childbirth in institutions and using clinics and home visits for providing prenatal and child health care and information and communication. In addition, women increasingly selected institutions where doctors were available to intervene when complications arose, although delivery continued to be managed largely by midwives. Deliveries in maternity homes and rural and cottage hospitals declined to 10 percent by 1957, and in 1960 only 5 percent of deliveries occurred in maternity homes.

During the 1960s and 1970s, 60 to 70 percent of live births had skilled attendance. Unfortunately, data on the types of institutions where childbirth took place are inadequate; therefore, it is not possible to analyze the pattern. However, in 1962 specialized obstetric services were available in 21 government institutions, and 16 percent of the deliveries took place in those institutions (Amarasinghe 1962).

During the 1980s and 1990s, the proportion of childbirth occurring in high-level institutions, where services of a consultant obstetri-

Table 18. Deliveries in the Private Sector, Sri Lanka, 1981–93

SECTOR	% DELIVERIES IN PRIVATE INSTITUTIONS	
	FAMILY HEALTH IMPACT SURVEY 1981	DEMOGRAPHIC AND HEALTH SURVEY 1993
Estate	0	0.3
Rural	2.0	2.8
Urban	8.7	23.0
All	2.9	6.5

Note: "All" is the weighted average of the different sectors.
Sources: Vidyasagara 1983; Sri Lanka, Department of Census and Statistics 1995.

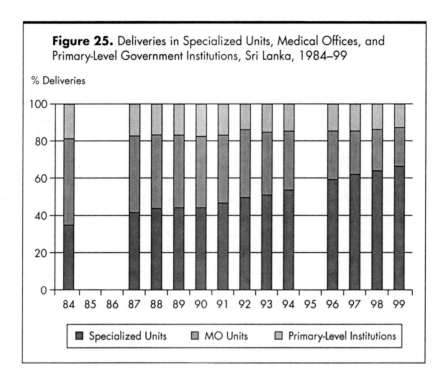

Figure 25. Deliveries in Specialized Units, Medical Offices, and Primary-Level Government Institutions, Sri Lanka, 1984–99

cian were available, increased from 36 percent in 1984 to 66 percent in 1999. In contrast, childbirth in institutions that had only a medical officer without further qualifications in obstetrics decreased from 46 to 22 percent, and those in primary care institutions decreased from 18 to 12 percent (figure 25). Delivery at home attended by a midwife declined from 9 percent in 1970 to 2 percent in 1995. With the increase in the number of private hospital beds, particularly in the urban areas, the percentage of deliveries in these institutions also increased (table 18).

Causes of Maternal Death

The relative contribution of different factors and interventions in reducing the MMR has been a topic of much interest. The design of this study and the types of data available do not support any conclusions about the contribution of different factors in the Sri Lankan context. However, given the current knowledge of the causal pathways of the major clinical causes of maternal death, a review of trends in causes of maternal deaths in Sri Lanka, in conjunction with the changing pattern of childbirth, provides valuable insights.

Nationwide data on causes of maternal death are not available for the 1930s, when rates of skilled attendance were below 30 percent. However, an analysis of the causes of maternal deaths that occurred at the De Soysa maternity home in Colombo between 1933 and 1938 showed that "associated or inter-current diseases" caused 54 percent of all fatalities (Wickramasuriya 1939, p. 87). Wickramasuriya (1939) commented that these data constitute "definite evidence of the poor standards of health of the women in the country" (p. 88). The important associated diseases were identified as ankylostomiasis (hookworm), malaria, nontuberculosis respiratory diseases, chronic enteritis, and dysentery. Ankylostomiasis was perceived as the "most important single factor in maternal and fetal mortality" (Wickramasuriya 1939, p. 91). Age- and sex-specific mortality due to ankylostomiasis and malaria both indicated a greater vulnerability of women, especially for those ages 15 to 49. Fernando (1994) concluded that control of these infections was therefore more favorable to women.

Maternal deaths due to hypertensive disease and sepsis show a marked decrease during the 1940s (figure 26). The decline in deaths due to these two causes match the fall in MMR and accounted for a greater proportion of the decline (table 19). During the 10-year period to 1950, skilled attendance increased substantially to 58 percent of births, with about 40 percent of the skilled attendance being at the home of the client (table 17). Attendance at antenatal clinics was high. Midwives became more abundant and accessible. The number of midwives in relation to the number of births improved considerably, for an average of one midwife for every 163 births in 1950 (table 20). As described earlier, malaria control also was successful during this period, and sanitation and nutrition are believed to have improved greatly.

Deaths due to hemorrhage did not show a significant decline during this period. Blood transfusion facilities were available in the

General Hospital Colombo and a few hospitals close to Colombo beginning in 1948. In the 1950s, O-positive blood was available in the provincial hospitals. During the 1940–50 period, most institutional deliveries took place in the smaller hospitals, and access to blood transfusion during emergencies was probably limited.

The major decline in the proportion of deaths due to hemorrhage occurred from the 1950s to the 1970s (table 19 and figure 27). Although the pattern of place of delivery continued to change, new measures and interventions were also introduced. In addition to the increase in births with skilled attendants in institutional settings, access to specialized services in most secondary and tertiary care hospitals increased. This shift was accompanied by the development and spread of blood transfusion services, and field midwives were allowed

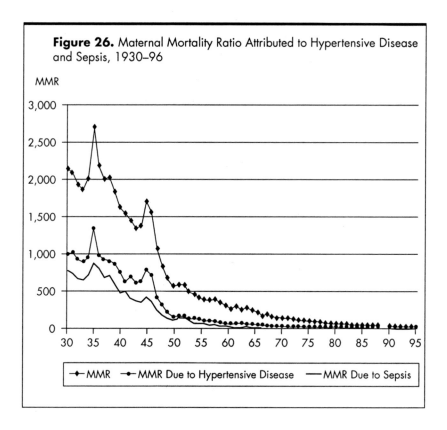

Figure 26. Maternal Mortality Ratio Attributed to Hypertensive Disease and Sepsis, 1930–96

to use oral ergometrine without direct supervision starting in 1978. Public health nursing sisters (PHNS) and nursing sisters[6] working in the smaller institutions that had no medical officers, were permitted

Table 19. Decline in Cause-Specific Maternal Mortality Ratio, Sri Lanka, 1942–52, 1955–70, and 1980–96

YEAR	MMR			
	ALL CAUSES	SEPSIS	HYPERTENSIVE DISEASE	HEMORRHAGE
1942	1,445	408	696	129
1952	580	143	161	113
1955	405	72	123	91
1970	145	20	37	45
1980	65	3	23	12
1996	24	0.3	0.6	8
	PERCENTAGE DECLINE			
1942–52	60	65	77	12
1955–70	64	72	70	51
1980–96	64	91	97	32

Source: Authors' calculations based on data from the Registrar General's Department.

Table 20. Development of Government-Employed Birth Attendants, Sri Lanka, 1930–95

YEAR	LIVE BIRTHS PER GOVERNMENT MIDWIFE	POPULATION PER 1,000 GOVERNMENT DOCTORS	GOVERNMENT NURSES PER GOVERNMENT DOCTOR	SPECIALIST OBSTETRICIANS IN GOVERNMENT HOSPITALS PER 100,000 LIVE BIRTHS
1930	405	15.4	—	—
1935	219	—	—	—
1940	—	14.8	—	—
1945	186	—	—	—
1950	163	11.4	1.7	—
1955	157	9.2	2.3	—
1960	143	8.4	2.8	6.6
1965	—	7.5	2.4	—
1970	—	6.5	2.9	—
1975	—	6.4	2.7	—
1980	125	7.2	3.3	14.0
1985	85	7.4	3.8	15.0
1990	68	7.0	3.7	20.0
1995	51	4.0	2.9	23.0

— Not available.
Source: Authors' compilation of data from various sources.

to use intramuscular ergometrine. The Ministry of Health (MOH) circulated detailed guidelines on when to use ergometrine. In 1962, the National Blood Transfusion Service was formed and a hospital-based regional blood banking service commenced; by 1994 there were 50 regional blood banks. Fresh-frozen plasma was available at the district level beginning in 1983, and all districts were covered by 1993. Between 1983 and 1995, blood components became available in all provincial and base hospitals (De Zoysa, informant interview).

Maternal deaths due to abortion have steadily declined, from 22.9 per 100,000 live births in 1936 to 1.5 per 100,000 live births in 1996. Maternal mortality figures over the years indicate that abortion contributes to approximately 10 percent of the reported deaths (Senevi-

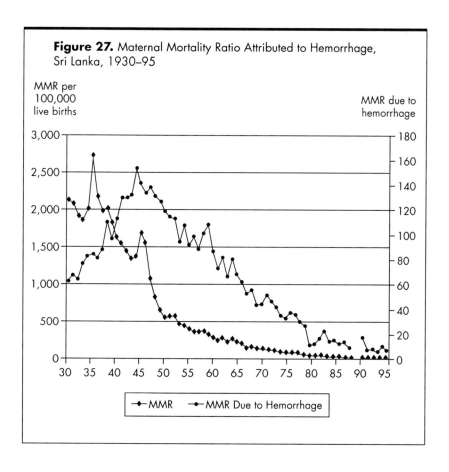

Figure 27. Maternal Mortality Ratio Attributed to Hemorrhage, Sri Lanka, 1930–95

ratne and Rajapaksa 2000). Rodrigo and others (n.d.) used multiple sources to identify causes of maternal death and found that induced abortions and puerperal sepsis each contributed 8 percent to maternal deaths.

Fertility and Maternal Mortality

The relationship of fertility to MMR is a topic of ongoing interest among policymakers and others. In Sri Lanka, initiation of family planning activities commenced in 1953, when a group of social workers supported by the government formed the Family Planning Association. In 1965 the government initiated islandwide family planning services. These services were incorporated into the MOH's field MCH services and reached the community through the PHM, whose role was well accepted in the community. The fact that family planning was introduced through the MCH package as a means of improving maternal and infant health contributed much to the acceptance of family planning in the country. The changes in contraceptive prevalence are shown in table 21.

It took 20 years—from 1952 to 1972—for the total fertility rate (TFR) to decline from 5.2 to 4.1. The next 10 years, however, it fell to 3.2, and in the next 14 years it fell to 2.1 (figure 28).

No major fall in TFR occurred during the 1950s and early 1960s. The limited decline in fertility from 1953 to 1963 has been attrib-

Table 21. Contraceptive Prevalence Rate, Sri Lanka, 1975–2000

METHOD	YEAR				
	1975[a]	1982[b]	1987[c]	1993[c]	2000[d]
Modern	18.8	30.4	40.6	43.7	49.5
Traditional	13.2	24.5	21.1	22.4	21.3
Any	32.0	54.9	61.7	66.1	70.8

Note: Modern methods of family planning consist of oral contraceptives, intrauterine devices, injectables such as Depo-Provera (depo medoxy progesterone acetate), condom, Norplant, and male and female sterilization. Traditional methods include safe period, withdrawal, and other practices.
Sources: [a] Alam and Cleland 1981; [b] Sri Lanka, Department of Census and Statistics 1983; [c] Sri Lanka, Department of Census and Statistics 1995; [d] Sri Lanka, Department of Census and Statistics 2001.

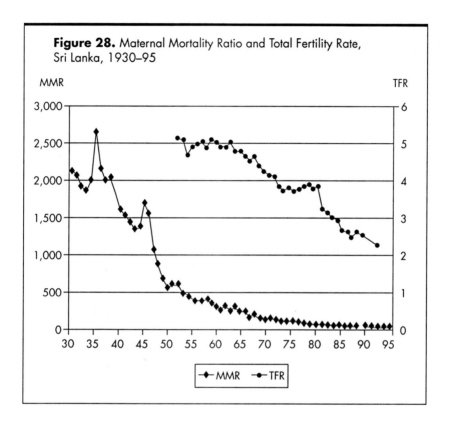

Figure 28. Maternal Mortality Ratio and Total Fertility Rate, Sri Lanka, 1930–95

uted mainly to increasing age at marriage and to changes in the age structure of the female population (Jayawardene and Selvaratnam 1967). Increasing participation of women in education led to increased age at marriage; the singulate mean age at marriage for women in education increased from 22.1 in 1963 to 25.1 in 1975, an increase of 3 years during a 12-year period (Perera and others 1999). The percentage of never-married 20- to 24-year-olds also rose steadily, from 30 percent in 1946 to 60 percent in 1975—a doubling in one generation (Dissanayake 1999).

From 1962–75, the greatest decline in fertility occurred among women ages 25 to 29, but in the late 1970s and early 1980s, fertility for women ages 25 and older decreased rapidly, resulting in a reduction in the high-risk pregnancies found in older age groups and high-parity pregnancies (figure 29). From 1962 onward, a continuous

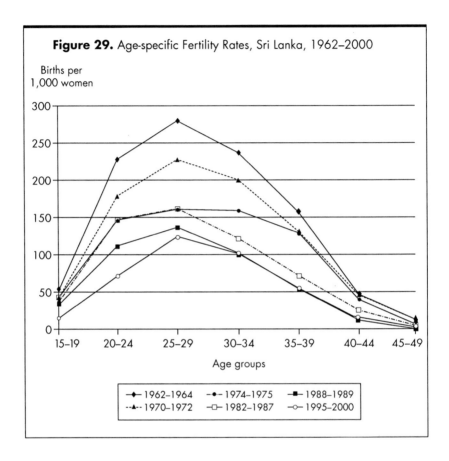

Figure 29. Age-specific Fertility Rates, Sri Lanka, 1962–2000

decline in fertility has occurred in all age groups. This reduction has been attributed to the proportion of females who get married and to changes in marital fertility. The proportion of the decline attributed to the latter cause increased from 41 percent in 1963–71 (Alam and Cleland 1981) to 54 percent in 1971–75. Retherford and Rele (1989) attributed 60 percent of the decline in TFR from 1960–84 to reduction in marital fertility. Although the marital fertility decline in Sri Lanka preceded the family planning program (Caldwell and others 1987), diffusion of modern methods of contraception undoubtedly resulted in the fertility decline since the 1970s.

The effects of the fertility decline among older women are reflected in the steeper decline in maternal mortality in the older age

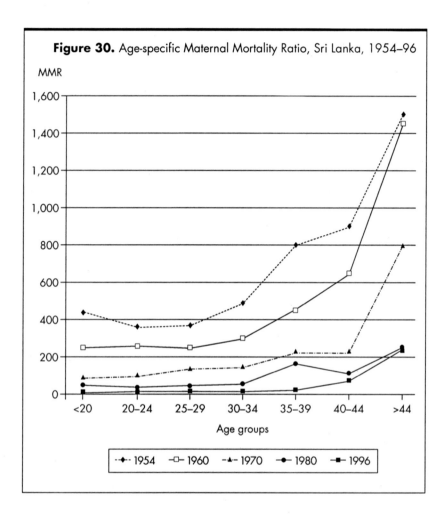

Figure 30. Age-specific Maternal Mortality Ratio, Sri Lanka, 1954–96

groups (figure 30). It was estimated that if all births to women older than age 35 had been prevented, a 27 percent reduction in maternal deaths in the period 1962–63 would have occurred (Wright 1969).

Development of Maternal and Child Health Services

The present day allopathic health services of Sri Lanka evolved from the Military and Estate Medical Services introduced by the British. A

Civil Medical Department was established in 1857 (Wickramasinghe 1949), and in the decades preceding independence the government laid the foundation for a national health service. Many policy decisions made during this period had far-reaching consequences.

Early Steps

From the inception of a national health service, the government assumed responsibility for providing health care. Policymakers recognized that preventive and curative care and health promotion needed to be integrated. As early as 1926, curative and preventive services were brought under one office, that of the director of Medical and Sanitary Services. This policy predated by several decades the international recognition of the importance of close linkages between preventive and curative services, particularly in the field of maternal health (Chellappah 1949).

The development of MCH services under the Western allopathic system of medicine can be traced back to the establishment of the De Soysa Lying in Home (in Colombo, the capital of Sri Lanka) in 1879. An important function of the institution from its inception was providing training in midwifery. Registration of midwives was made compulsory in 1887. In 1902 a maternal and child health department was created within the municipality of Colombo; an organized effort to provide field maternal health services commenced in 1906, when the services of trainee midwives were used for maternal care within the municipality. The first antenatal clinic was held at the De Soysa Lying in Home in 1921 (Fernando 1996).

Health Infrastructure

The establishment of the first Health Unit in 1926 was an important landmark in the development of the health care system of the country. This system remains the cornerstone of the field health services even today.

Health Units. The Health Unit system resulted in the expansion of delivery of MCH services to a broader population. The system provided both institutional and domiciliary care for the mother and child. Clinic services were provided through health centers or field antenatal clinics located within the community in proximity to the people. PHMs were responsible for the care of all pregnant women in their area. Their responsibilities included early identification and registration of all pregnant mothers, provision of regular antenatal care, domiciliary and clinic care, identification and intervention for women at risk, planning a place of confinement to ensure safe delivery, assistance at home delivery when needed, and care of mothers and newborn babies during the postnatal period.

Initially, the expansion of the Health Unit system was slow because it was perceived to be too expensive. However, evaluation of the impact of the disastrous malaria epidemic in the mid-1930s showed that areas that had Health Units fared better than those without them. Subsequently, expansion of the system accelerated, and by 1948 the entire island was covered. Simultaneously, the training of government midwives was stepped up, and despite high fertility rates, the number of births per midwife decreased from 400 in 1930 to 163 by 1950. Thus, the 1930s and 1940s can be viewed as a germinal period in the expansion of maternal care.

A Health Unit headed by a medical officer of health serves the population of a defined geographic area. Each Health Unit is further subdivided into PHM areas, which are the smallest working units in the field health care system and serve a population of 3,000 to 5,000. This system emphasizes preventive and health promotion services at the community level delivered by a medical officer and a team of field health workers. With the increase in the number of Health Units came rapid growth in the number of health centers that provided antenatal and child health activities (table 22).

Islandwide Diffusion of Services. A dominant feature of the health services in Sri Lanka from an early stage has been the diffusion of services throughout the country. The National Health Manpower Study reported that "a health care delivery unit can be found, on the average, not further than 0.8 miles from any home in the country and free of charge western type health care services are available within 3 miles of a patient's home" (Simeonov 1975, p. 163).

Table 22. Development of Maternal-Health-Care-Related Infrastructure, Sri Lanka, 1931–95

YEAR	HOSPITALS PER 100,000 POPULATION	BEDS PER 100,000 POPULATION	HEALTH CENTERS PER 100,000 LIVE BIRTHS
1931	2.9	182a	30
1937	2.0	204	45
1940	—	—	195
1947	2.7	243	211
1950	3.4	260	230
1955	3.1	281	236
1960	2.9	301	247
1965	2.6	300	271
1970	2.6	302	—
1975	2.6	293	—
1980	2.6	287	—
1985	2.5	245	—
1990	2.1	248	—
1995	2.4	263	—

— Not available.
a1932 data
Source: Authors' compilation of data from various sources.

Network of Institutions. The field health services are well supported by a strong institutional network throughout the country. The institutional network within each province is structured to form a three-tiered system. At the apex, there are a number of tertiary teaching and specialist institutions, as well as the provincial or general hospitals, which have a range of specialist services, and a few base hospitals that offer, at a minimum, the four major specialties: medicine, surgery, pediatrics and obstetrics and gynecology. The next or secondary level comprises a number of district hospitals and peripheral units, where the services of doctors are available. The peripheral units remain the lowest level of institution in the health care network where services of doctors are available. They are equipped to provide general inpatient services in addition to maternity care. At the third or primary level are rural hospitals, cottage hospitals, and maternity homes, some of which are associated with central dispensaries, which also provide maternity services and are served by registered and assistant medical practitioners (table 23). All the primary-level institutions in a given area are under the supervision of the medical officer of health for the area.

Table 23. Categories of Institution, Sri Lanka

LEVEL	TYPES OF INSTITUTION	SERVICES AVAILABLE	
Tertiary	Teaching hospitals Specialist maternity hospitals	Range of specialist services Specialist obstetric and gynecological services	Laboratory, radiological facilities, blood transfusion services, operating theaters, and anesthetic facilities
	Provincial or general hospitals Base hospitals	Range of specialist services Four basic specialties at a minimum	
Secondary	District hospitals Peripheral units	Nonspecialist medical officers	Indoor and outdoor facilities General inpatient as well as maternity care Blood (in large district hospitals)
Primary	Cottage hospitals, rural hospitals, maternity homes (may be associated with a central dispensary, where outpatient facilities are available)	Registered/assistant medical practitioners Midwifery-qualified sisters Midwives	General inpatient as well as maternity care IV fluids, plasma expanders

Note: An assistant medical practitioner (AMP) is a category of health professional that is trained for 3 years, in contrast to a 5-year MBBS curriculum. Entry criteria are also lower: After a specified number of years of service and examination, AMPs get promoted to registered medical practitioners (RMP).
Source: Authors.

In 1930, a total of 112 government hospitals were functioning in all nine provinces of the country. There were two provincial hospitals in Kandy and Galle in addition to the general hospital in Colombo. The postwar years brought a rapid expansion of government health institutions, which was facilitated by the external resources accumulated during the war years. By 1948 the number of hospitals had increased to 247, including five provincial hospitals; in 2 years, 4 more provincial hospitals were added, and the total number of institutions increased to 263.

Secondary- and tertiary-level institutions for maternity care expanded during the 1950s. A second tertiary-level maternity hospital opened in 1950, and by 1954, 9 provincial and 11 base hospitals

all provided specialized obstetric care in addition to the two maternity hospitals in Colombo (De Silva 1956). The concept of a "peripheral unit" with a doctor in charge was introduced during this period,
and women gained greater access to facilities served by a doctor.

The number of hospitals continued to increase in the 1960s. A
characteristic of this increase was the expansion of the number of secondary and tertiary institutions where specialist or nonspecialist doctors were available. The number of provincial and base hospitals
where specialist obstetric services were available increased by 30 percent between 1964 and 1983, and the number of district hospitals and
peripheral units where services of nonspecialist doctors were available
increased by 41 percent. Cottage hospitals, rural hospitals, and maternity homes increased by only 9 percent during the same period.

The number of government institutions with maternity services
increased to 490 by the end of 1996, and the countrywide network
comprised 2 special maternity hospitals, 45 institutions where services of specialist obstetricians were available, 266 district hospitals and
peripheral units where doctors were available, and 177 units where
registered medical practitioners or midwifery-qualified sisters were
in charge (Sri Lanka Ministry of Health 1997).

Although the total number of institutions increased, this growth
did not keep pace with the increase in population, and the number of
institutions per head of population decreased from 1950 onward.
The bed strength per population increased up to 1970, and then it,
too, started to decline (table 22).

Transport of Mothers with Complications and Emergencies. The ambulance service, which was started in 1926 with 2 ambulances, had only
12 ambulances in 1948 but rapidly expanded to a fleet of 67 ambulances by 1950. More important, all provincial hospitals were provided with three to five ambulances each, as were all major district
hospitals and "less important hospitals situated in the more remote
parts where other means of transportation are not easily available"
(Wickramasinghe 1952, p. 272).

In the absence of an ambulance or other form of official transportation, and in situations in which it is not possible or feasible to
call for an ambulance, field health staff are authorized to hire private

transportation for emergency referral. In the 1930s–50s, this transportation might take the form of a bullock cart or a buggy in remote rural areas. In recent years, it might be a taxi or a private vehicle. In such cases, the money paid for the transport is reimbursed by the MOH. According to the key informants, the system functions well, and any expenses incurred are normally reimbursed within a reasonable length of time (Fernando, informant interview).

One situation that may be a barrier to access is the case of clients with obstetric complications who have not yet made contact with a PHM or any other part of the health system. Although they noted this barrier, the key informants felt that in light of the relatively short distances involved in Sri Lanka, even in the most remote parts of the country, women who needed and sought help with referral would normally be able to identify a means of transportation from within her community.

Development of Health Personnel

Health planners recognized that a mixture of health personnel was necessary to improve access to care, and the training of different categories of health staff was addressed systematically.

Training of Midwives. Formal training in midwifery began in 1879 and was limited to trained nurses. Legislation enacted in 1897 required persons who practiced midwifery to be trained in accordance with a prescribed curriculum and their names placed on a midwives' register maintained by the Sri Lanka Medical Council. Registration of midwives was made mandatory and enhanced the quality of midwifery early on. This professionalization of midwifery is considered an important development. Entry for training as a midwife required at least 8 years of school education; the requirement later increased to 11 years and is currently 13 years. The training is carried out in accordance with a curriculum that emphasizes hands-on clinical training, including strict adherence to defined procedures. Until 1926 midwives functioned only in hospitals, and the training was entirely hospital based and conducted by nursing tutors and by consultant obstetricians.

The present system of 18 months of training commenced in 1936. At the inception of this system the trainees spent their first 12 months at the De Soysa Lying in Home and the next 6 months at the Health Unit in Kalutara (Gunesekara 1938). Currently, the first year is spent in a school of nursing; the next 6 months of training takes place in a field training area. To qualify for the final examination, students must observe 10 normal deliveries, conduct 20 normal deliveries under supervision, and assist in 5 abnormal deliveries as well as look after 25 normal babies and 10 sick babies. Students maintain logbooks that must be signed by the supervisor attesting to satisfactory completion of the required tasks. The importance accorded to the training is evidenced by documentary evidence of participation of the deputy director of Public Health Services and consultant obstetricians as examiners and their recommendations regarding curriculum and teaching approaches. On successful completion of training, a PHM-trainee is awarded a certificate, is registered with the Medical Council, and is appointed to either a hospital or Health Unit as a PHM. On graduation, PHMs are awarded a badge, which is highly prestigious. During earlier decades, midwifery was a highly sought-after profession because "there were few alternatives for educated girls" (de Silva, de Costa, and others, informant interviews). Midwifery training for nurses (see below) has similar clinical requirements for completing practical clinical tasks.

The Public Health Midwife. PHMs have become the cornerstone of the Health Unit system. They serve a population of 3,000 to 5,000 within a clearly defined area and live in the village, usually in rented rooms. The Ministry of Health has built living quarters for midwives in a few locations. Families who have space to rent are those who are well known in the village; their status helps the PHM gain acceptance and respectability within the village (Nimal Vidyasagara, informant interview). PHMs visit the homes of pregnant women, register them for care, persuade them to attend antenatal clinics, and work beside the doctor who conducts the antenatal clinics. The clinics (referred to as field health centers) are often in premises rented on a part-time basis from a resident in the community or in a peripheral institution, such as a maternity home. Thus, PHMs not only provide services at the community level but also link the mother and child to the next level of care, the health center. During childbirth, the PHM provides skilled attendance at home. The PHM has come to be accepted by the community not only as a government functionary but also as a health professional in her own right (box 4).

The Nurse–Midwife. Formal training in nursing commenced in Sri Lanka with the establishment of a nurses' training school at the General Hospital Colombo in 1878, and regulations regarding duties of nurses were framed the following year. These early attempts experienced difficulty in attracting "suitable pupils" for training and resulted in the recruitment of nursing nuns. In 1881 a school to train nurses in midwifery was established in the De Soysa Lying in Home under the supervision of the matron. The training initially lasted 3 months and was later extended to 6 months. In 1905, another nursing school was established in Kandy, and by 1957 Sri Lanka had a total of eight schools of nursing. Gradually, the nursing services were extended to all hospitals to become an integral part of the health care system. During the early period the duration of training varied from 1 year in Colombo to 2 years in Kandy. Currently, nurses undergo a basic training of 3 years. To be registered as a midwife, a further 6 months of midwifery training is required. Promotion to ward sister requires successful completion of 1 year of training in a postbasic school of nursing. A PHNS has a further 6 months of field training in addition to midwifery and postbasic training.

Supervision and Support. Midwife training equips trainees with skills for self-assessment that are supported by a system of record keeping. The supervisory officers in the field are the Supervising PHMs, who answer to the PHNS; both positions report to the medical officer of health. Procedures for such supervision are specified and are supportive, rather than punitive, although punitive measures are taken if the need arises. The midwife sends standardized monthly and quarterly reports, or "returns," to the MOH of the different services she has provided. Returns from all midwives falling within a PHNS area are collated by the respective PHNS. This step provides an opportunity to assess the work of the midwives. The monthly conference of all staff under each medical officer of health is an opportunity to discuss problems and provide refresher education as well as to expose midwives to current knowledge. This system of supervision has been in existence from the inception of the Health Unit system.

Box 4. We Are Proud of Our Public Health Midwives

"During 1960–65 I participated in village health programs which gave me good insight into the problems of rural people. Maternal health services were very popular. PHMs were highly respected. Dressed in their white sarees with blue borders they looked like angels as they moved around the villages. I realized that one of their problems was transport and I managed to get them bicycles. This greatly improved the coverage of the services they provided."

Obeyesekere, minister of health during the 1970s

"Supervisory PHMs provided excellent grassroots level support and encouragement. Discipline was very good, and PHMs were very dedicated to their work. Monthly meetings at the office of the medical officer of health were a regular feature during which problems were reviewed and supplies given to PHMs. PHMs were well respected and their advice sought by the women in the area. They would secretively ask for contraceptives from the PHMs although family planning was not openly accepted at that time."

Fernando, district medical officer in the 1960s

"Fifty percent to 70 percent of PHMs are absolutely fantastic. Surveys show that the PHM is one of the happiest groups of workers we have studied. The PHM is well trained, placed in a nice system that is highly supportive, and has a little universe where her work is well defined. She

Box 4. (continued)

knows her clientele very well and has avenues (monthly meetings) to ventilate her problems."

Wijemanne, UNICEF program officer, 1970–2001

"The PHM is a category of staff that has done excellent work and should receive major credit for the low MMR in our country. Even today when most women deliver in hospital, she continues to visit the mothers in their homes. Her advice is sound and well respected, as I know from the personal experience of my own daughter-in-law."

Dr. Akkarakkuruppu Mudiyanselage Lokubardara Beligaswatte, director general of health, 1998–2002

Midwives working in hospital settings are supervised by the nurse–midwife and sisters or matrons in charge of the institution and the medical officers. In an emergency the midwives working in the field can directly call on either the PHNS or the medical officer of health. All small institutions with no qualified doctor falling within a Health Unit area are supervised by the medical officer of health. In an emergency midwives and nurses working in such institutions can call the medical officer of health or directly transfer the patient to a higher-level institution.

The number of midwives has steadily increased over time, and the number of mothers in each midwife's caseload has steadily decreased (table 20).

Training of Doctors. A medical school had been established in Colombo by 1870, and midwifery training was introduced to the medical curriculum in 1915. With the opening of a second medical school in 1961, the number of doctors registered with the Sri Lanka Medical Council increased from 29 per 100,000 population in 1961 to 48 per 100,000 population in 1979, but the proportion of doctors employed by the government did not reflect this increase. In 1960 the ratio in government service was 12 per 100,000 population, which increased slowly to 15 per 100,000 in 1970 and jumped to 30 per 100,000 by 1996.

Specialist Obstetricians. As early as 1930, the De Soysa Lying in Home had the services of an assistant obstetrician. By 1953 the number of specialist obstetricians had increased to 23. In 1962 specialized obstetric services were available in 21 government institutions, and 24 obstetricians were in government service (Amarasinghe 1962). By 1967 the number of obstetricians had doubled to 50. The ratio of obstetricians to 100,000 live births increased from 6.6 in 1962 to 13.5 in 1967 and rose to 24 in 1996. The number of specialists has rapidly increased in recent times.

Management of Maternal and Child Health Programs

Many infrastructure developments within the MOH in the 1950s had an impact on maternal health. In the mid-1950s, a health education division was formed and the post of medical officer of maternal and child health (MOMCH) was created; this person was responsible for coordinating all MCH services in a district. Another important development in MCH services was the formation of the Maternal and Child Health Bureau in 1968, which had a director in charge of all MCH work on the island.

Management Strategies for Improved Maternal Care. In the first phase of maternal mortality decline, the emphasis was on making services accessible to the majority of the population, a goal that was achieved through distributing a large number of small institutions in all parts of the island. The goal was to improve antenatal coverage and detection and early referral of complications. The importance accorded to maternal health services is reflected in the detailed reports on field and institutional services provided in the reports of the DHS at the time.

For example, difficulties in transporting patients were recognized early by the government. The report of the DHS in 1951 stated that the "aim of the department has been to establish throughout the island an ambulance service which with the aid of telephone facilities, will provide quick and safe transport for the sick, from their homes to the smaller hospitals or from the latter to the larger hospitals" (Wickramasinghe 1952, p. 272).

The second phase involved intensive monitoring of the field MCH program and included the appointment of a MOMCH for each district in 1961. The Maternal and Child Health Bureau formed in 1968 was renamed the Family Health Bureau (FHB) in 1973. Field reporting systems were reorganized, and the director of maternal and child health (D/MCH) collated all data on MCH and family planning services. This approach resulted in intensive and regular program review and supervision along with inservice training programs to address deficiencies. In the late 1970s the FHB produced a manual for midwives, which was printed in Sinhala, Tamil, and English. The effective reporting system and regular monitoring and evaluation no doubt contributed to the maintenance of high standards in MCH services.

With government acceptance of family planning as national policy in 1965, the MCH Bureau (later the FHB) was made the central organization responsible for family planning activities. Evaluation of MCH programs was also an important function of the MCH Bureau.

The third phase emphasized quality-of-care issues. The findings of maternal death inquiries were used to identify deficiencies in the system. The MOH developed essential drug and equipment lists for small hospitals as well as instruction circulars that were based on deficiencies identified at maternal death reviews. Clinical protocols have recently been developed and circulated to all institutions. Innovative approaches to linking consultant obstetricians in provincial or base hospitals with the peripheral services have been tried as measures for reducing the problem of overcrowded specialist units. Management decisions, such as appointing two obstetricians to an institution, ensuring 24-hour ambulance access, and making blood more widely available for transfusion, are other recent initiatives.

Maternal Death Monitoring. The DHS reports provide evidence that a maternal death investigation procedure was in existence during the late 1950s. During this period, the medical officer of health of the area, using a prescribed form, investigated all maternal deaths. Relatives of the deceased, the PHM of the area, and hospital staff were interviewed, and relevant records were examined. Follow-up action was left to the local medical officer of health and the head of the relevant institution. In 1959 a committee was established to investigate maternal mortality, and an amended investigation form was developed, field tested, and used beginning in 1962 (Herath-Guneratne 1965).

In August 1968 the Association of Obstetricians and Gynaecologists of Ceylon held a seminar on maternal mortality and submitted to the MOH a memorandum with recommendations for the reduction of maternal mortality. They suggested that an "advisory committee" of the association study all maternal deaths on the island, that the data should be considered confidential, and that a quarterly or biannual report should be submitted to the DHS. They further suggested that a committee including officers of the MOH and the association should study these reports (Association of Obstetricians and Gynaecologists of Ceylon 1969).

During the early 1970s a circular instructed hospitals to implement a standard procedure to look for avoidable causes of death; it was not implemented in all hospitals or districts, however. In some districts, the process involved only the institution concerned, whereas in others, the district health staff also participated. By 1977, implementation became more stringent; follow up was systematic and included management at the district and central levels.

Maternal death investigation in the present form commenced in 1989. All maternal deaths are reported to the D/FHB, the provincial director of health services (PDHS), and the deputy provincial director of health services (DPDHS). If a death occurs in an institution, the head of the institution is responsible for reporting the death; if it occurs in the field, the medical officer of health has this responsibility.

All maternal deaths are investigated and reported on in a specified format within 7 days. Investigation of a maternal death is the responsibility of the head of the institution. Participants comprise the head of the institution, the consultant obstetrician, the medical officer who attended to the deceased, the nurse or sister in charge of the labor room, the MOMCH, and the medical officer of health of the area of residence of the mother. A report of the investigation is sent to the D/FHB and DPDHS. In addition to the institutional inquiry, a separate field investigation is carried out by the medical officer of health, the PHNS, and the PHM to examine care prior to admission. This is reported independently to the DPDHS as well as to the FHB. Deaths occurring in the field are investigated by the MOMCH and reported to the PDHS, DPDHS, and D/FHB.

In 1985, a formal system of maternal death review (audit) was introduced, which was inspired by the successful Extended Programme of Immunization (EPI) review programs. At their inception, the reviews occurred annually at the central level; these reviews were given high priority, as evidenced by the fact that the DGHS chaired the meetings. Currently, the reviews take place quarterly at the district level and annually at the national level. Participants in these reviews include the DGHS, provincial health administrators, the D/FHB, representatives of the College of Obstetricians and Gynecologists, community physicians, university academics, and heads of relevant institutions. At the reviews, each death is discussed not merely to find the cause of death but to analyze the circumstances of death. The "three delays" model is used to identify shortcomings: delay in deciding to seek medical care, delay in reaching a medical facility with adequate care, and delay in receiving quality care at the facility.

Participants have gradually accepted that the reviews are not a "fault-finding exercise" but a means of correcting quality-of-care issues. At the end of the review, specific corrective actions to be taken are identified, some of which the regional authorities can implement immediately. Issues identified include the need for training in obstetrics for medical officers before they are posted to hospitals where consultant services are not available, availability of plasma expanders (in smaller hospitals) and of blood (in the larger district hospitals), 24-hour coverage in specialist units, delays within the hospital, and vacancy of PHM posts in the area in which the death occurred.

Other key quality-of-care issues that have been identified as contributory factors in maternal deaths include bypassing of small hospitals and overcrowding of wards with specialist services, resulting in heavy workloads for obstetricians in specialist hospitals. As a result, clinical management protocols have been developed and circulated to all hospitals offering maternity services. The MOH and the College of Obstetricians and Gynecologists are planning and coordinating remedial measures, demonstrating another example of the close collaboration between health managers and clinical staff in Sri Lanka (Beligaswatte, Fernando, Jayathilake, and Senanayaka, informant interviews).

Implementation of Critical Health Policies

Review of the Sri Lankan experience suggests an evolutionary process that has several similarities with the Malaysian experience summarized in the previous chapter.

Foundations for Effective Maternal Health Care

Policies initiated during the latter half of the 19th century and the early 20th century laid the foundations for professional midwifery. Legislation governing the practice was enacted, training curricula and standards were established, and certification and registration of midwives began. Civil registration of births and deaths was governed by legislation, and maternal deaths were viewed with sufficient concern to warrant special reporting by the RG. Models for service delivery providing an integrated package of MCH care through clinics near the communities they served were developed and found to be feasible and popular. Most important, the PHM was established and accepted as the principal provider of maternity care at the community level.

Political and Policy Environment

The early gains in female education and the empowerment of women through the electoral process provided an environment that sustained political and managerial commitment to improving maternal health. Moreover, the political philosophies provided the framework for reaching out to remote and disadvantaged communities. Political commitment to and societal expectations of health and education services to be provided free of charge to the entire population served to remove financial barriers to maternity care.

Improved Access

The decades of the 1930s through the 1950s could be characterized as focused on improving geographic access to health care. The health service infrastructure was expanded, and human resources were developed pragmatically and rapidly. High-level management attention ensured that strict training standards were maintained during the period of rapid expansion. A strong supervisory structure ensured attention to quality during the expansion phase.

Narrowing of Interdistrict Differentials in the Maternal Mortality Ratio

The impact of the efforts to improve access is evident. Rodrigo (1987) analyzed the district MMRs for the periods 1962–64, 1970–72, and 1980–82 and reported that every district achieved considerable reduction in MMR during the period and that interdistrict variation was considerably narrowed. The magnitude of the reduction was observed to be greater in the areas that had higher mortality in 1962–64. This finding suggests accelerated improvements in health services and socioeconomic conditions in the less developed districts of the country.

Similar Utilization of Maternity Services by All Income Groups

Another critical feature of the childbirth pattern was that similar proportions of women from low- and high-income groups gave birth in institutions. Vidyasagara (1983) and Wickramasuriya (1939) analyzed data from the Family Health Impact Survey (table 24) and noted that "forty three percent of all births in government institutions were from the lower income group suggesting that government expenditure on health does reach the segment of population most in need" (p. 102).

Table 24. Place of Delivery by Monthly Family Income, Sri Lanka, 1982

	MONTHLY INCOME IN RUPEES			
PLACE OF DELIVERY	<300	300–599	600–999	1,000+
Home	25.5	22.4	8.6	6.6
Government institution	70.2	73.2	83.8	77.0
Private nursing home	1.4	1.7	5.7	16.4
Unknown	2.9	2.7	1.9	0.0
Total	100.0	100.0	100.0	100.0

Source: Vidyasagara 1983.

Special Efforts for Disadvantaged Groups

The "estate population" illustrates the pragmatic approach to identifying and addressing issues. The Family Health Impact Survey (Vidyasagara 1983 and Wickramasuriya 1939) showed that the place selected for childbirth was similar in urban and rural populations. However, the estate population differed in that more than 50 percent of deliveries took place in unsuitable rooms for safe childbirth. The government noted with concern that this pattern existed even in areas that had easy access to hospitals and maternity homes, and it began instituting measures to address the issue (table 25).

Policymakers recognized that the Indian Tamils living and working on the estates, who constituted about 6 percent of Sri Lanka's population, were less literate than the general population (81 versus 61 percent) and other disadvantaged populations. Political development after independence left them disenfranchised. Because this population was isolated within privately or foreign-owned estates, social change, including education and health, tended to bypass them. Hygiene was poor, and malnutrition was widespread. Often estate women delivered in line rooms that were unhygienic and unsuited for delivery and were attended to by untrained midwives. The employers were responsible for the provision of health services. Although government hospitals were located within estate areas, the cost of services provided by the state institutions had to be borne by the management in the plantation sector, and the estate population had limited access to the national system. Utilization of health ser-

Table 25. Place of Delivery by Sector, Sri Lanka, 1982

PLACE OF DELIVERY	SECTOR			
	URBAN	RURAL	ESTATE	ALL SECTORS
Home	11.1	19.7	51.1	21.2
Government institution	78.0	75.9	43.8	73.2
Private nursing home	8.7	2.0	0	2.9
Unknown	2.2	2.4	5.1	2.6
All places	100.0	100.0	100.0	100.0

Note: Columns may not add to 100 due to rounding.
Source: Vidyasagara 1983.

vices was further limited due to low levels of education, cultural beliefs, and the low status accorded to women in this community. Socioeconomic surveys, however, indicate that household incomes and calorie intake in the estate sector were marginally higher than in some of the poor areas in the nonestate sector (Gunatilleke 2000).

Following nationalization of the estates in 1972, the accumulated burden of providing services became the government's responsibility. Medical officers with transport facilities and supported by PHNSs were appointed to establish a network of estate polyclinics that would provide integrated MCH and family planning services to meet the needs of the estate population. Through this program, knowledge and skills of estate health staff were upgraded, and women were given paid leave by the management to attend the polyclinics, which were held on a fixed day each month. This initiative and its acceptance by the estate management set the stage for introducing additional preventive health care activities on estates. In 1980, the two government estate management agencies developed their own social development divisions and initiated a series of interventions to improve water and sanitation on the estates and to improve conditions during childbirth through training of midwives, improved referral, and transportation. In addition, labor rooms were upgraded (Vidyasagara 2001).

The impact of the changes on skilled attendance is evident. Between 1986 and 1997, the pattern of childbirth among estate women changed from 20 to 63 percent of deliveries in government hospitals, 42 to 29 percent in estate maternity units, and from 37 to 8 percent in the home. Seventy percent of the births in the 5 years preceding the 1993 Demographic and Health Survey received skilled attendance, and 17 percent of estate women are reported to have been attended by a traditional birth attendant; a further 13 percent were attended by a relative or neighbor, whereas in 1997 only 5.4 percent received untrained assistance at delivery. In the 1980s and 1990s a "remarkable improvement in social indicators" occurred in the estate sector (Gunatilleke 2000, p. 161). The crude death rate dropped from 15 per 1,000 population in 1980 to 6.5 in 1997, close to the level of the rest of the country. Infant mortality declined from about 82 per 1,000 live births to 24 per 1,000 during the same period. The MMR declined from 120 per 100,000 live births in 1985 to 90 per 100,000 in 1997.

Improved Quality of Care

During the 1960s and 1970s, good access to basic health care had been established, and the focus of attention was on the introduction of family planning, improving the quality of care, and introducing advances in obstetric management. Monitoring systems were continually strengthened, and maternal death investigations were used to fuel improved clinical and organizational management.

After 1977 government health policies changed. Although the government commitment to providing free health services to the public was maintained, it promoted growth of the private sector. Government doctors were allowed private practice, which stimulated expansion of the private sector. Furthermore, a degree of decentralization of health management and administration occurred in 1990. The demand for health services expanded with increasing awareness of their availability among the population.

A high ratio of human resources to population had been achieved, leading to much higher proportions of midwives and doctors in Sri Lanka than in Malaysia. Simultaneously, a shift of childbirth to higher level institutions occurred during the 1980s and 1990s. The Simeonov study (1975) demonstrated that a midwife in a hospital setting managed a much higher number of deliveries than her counterpart who managed deliveries in the community. However, key informants shared a remarkable consensus about the pivotal role of PHMs working in the community in Sri Lanka today. They asserted that they are largely responsible for sustaining community confidence and satisfaction in the health care system and for the continued improvement in maternal health status despite any perceived short-comings in the health care delivery system.

Health System Expenditures, Affordability, and Sustainability

Expenditures on Maternal Health

In the past 50 years, the health system in Sri Lanka has been trans-formed from a primarily government-funded health system to one that relies on a combination of government and direct household expenditures. The system can be characterized as remarkably effi-cient, considering the maternal health outputs achieved with rela-tively modest financial inputs.

As shown in figure 31, from 1950–99 expenditures on maternal health services consistently declined, from an average of 0.28 per-cent of GDP in the 1950s to 0.16 percent of GDP in the 1990s, averaging 0.23 percent for the whole period over the five decades. In this context, the steady decline in maternal mortality during the same period is most remarkable. Table 26 illustrates the trend in the recurrent, capital, and total cost components of maternal health expenditures for the decades from 1950 through 1999.

Although it was not possible to disaggregate expenditures by health service location (that is, hospital, maternity home, or PHM outreach services), the trends in health services utilization make it clear that an ever-increasing share of expenditures is directed at the hospital level, which in the 1960s accounted for 64 percent of total expenditures (Jones and Selvaratnam 1972).

One important explanation of the ability of the system to achieve decreasing levels of maternal mortality was the efficiency gains real-ized in the 1950s and 1960s. During this period, utilization rose and government funding declined, but the health system was neverthe-

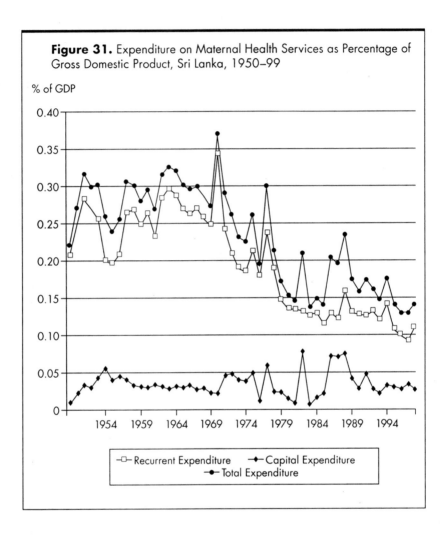

Figure 31. Expenditure on Maternal Health Services as Percentage of Gross Domestic Product, Sri Lanka, 1950–99

less able to sustain declines in maternal mortality by using inputs even more efficiently. "Public services delivered an increasing volume of services by halving unit costs during the 1950s to 1970s through using personnel and infrastructure more intensively" (Hsiao 2000, p. 61).

The effects of small entitlements on the morale of the midwife teams was certainly significant. They became recognized and respected in the communities (Beligaswatte, informant interview), an out-

Table 26. Maternal Health Care Expenditures, Sri Lanka, 1950–99

	% GDP			
	EXPENDITURES ON MATERNAL HEALTH CARE			TOTAL GOVERNMENT HEALTH EXPENDITURES
DECADE	RECURRENT	CAPITAL	TOTAL	
1950s	0.24	0.04	0.28	1.95
1960s	0.27	0.03	0.30	2.12
1970s	0.22	0.04	0.26	1.81
1980s	0.13	0.04	0.18	1.47
1990s	0.12	0.03	0.16	1.53
1950–99	0.20	0.04	0.23[a]	1.79

Note: Data may not sum to totals because of rounding.
[a]Data does not sum to total due to differences in the number of observations for recurrent and capital expenditures.
Source: Authors' compilation of data from various sources.

come that was important and motivated them to work hard. A number of the key informants repeated the theme: "The midwife of the bygone era was very dedicated" (Fernando, informant interview).

Underlying the reduction in government expenditures was the gradual reduction, in real terms, of the salaries of the health workers providing and supporting maternal health care. During the 50 years of this study, the salary of the staff providing maternal health services accounted for more than half of the total recurrent expenditures; the total expenditures on maternal health services are therefore sensitive to changes in salary rates and related expenses. Salaries expressed in terms of GDP per capita have declined significantly. This trend was confirmed in discussions with the key informants of the study. Although the negative impact of the reduction in real salaries on the motivation of the health workers is undeniable, the trend has led to an increased economic efficiency of the health system, which certainly contributed to its ability to provide care to an ever-increasing number of people.

Another factor that might have contributed to the ability of the system to achieve the decreases in maternal mortality despite falling public expenditures was the emerging role of the private sector. Between 1930 and 1950, primary health care services, including PHM outreach services, were gradually introduced throughout the country, funded entirely by government funds. This growth was

Table 27. Public and Private Health Services, Sri Lanka, 1953–96

YEAR	SOURCE OF NATIONAL HEALTH EXPENDITURES (%)	
	PUBLIC	PRIVATE
1953	62	38
1980	57	43
1990	46	54
1996	50	50

Source: Hsiao 2000.

accompanied by a gradual increase in the demand for these primary health care services as households learned about their nature and availability. The ability of the system to cope with the increasing demand in recent years was aided by the growth in utilization of private sector services, which provided care to an increasing share of the population that was able and willing to pay for them, as shown in table 27. The declining real wages of government health workers certainly had an impact on the availability of private care, because the government workers sought to maintain or increase their real incomes by working in the private sector after hours. The demand for services by a proportion of clients was transferred from the public to the private sector, thus reducing the demand for publicly provided outpatient care. Inpatient care remains predominantly public.

Affordability

Throughout the history of Sri Lanka, the health of its people has been a major concern to governments; services were therefore provided to ensure the well-being of vulnerable groups, such as mothers, children, and the aged, even during the reign of ancient kings (Seneviratne and Rajapaksa 2000). This policy has continued to the present day, and Sri Lanka has an extraordinarily high level of government commitment to and popular support for the welfare state, including support for universal free access to health care. So strong is the support and so politically sensitive is the topic that user fees will not be officially debated in a public forum (Hsiao 2000).

To assess the affordability of health services from a client perspective, this study examined client charges associated with maternal care, including antenatal care, normal delivery care, emergency obstetric care, and postpartum care. In evaluating charges, consideration was given to any fees related to health services and the purchase of drugs and supplies as well as to other associated expenditures, such as transportation, including transport involved in emergency referral.

User Fees

As early as 1903, the MOH had instituted a policy of implementing progressive user fees for health services, which were based on client income (De Silva and others 1997). According to the *Administration Report* of the director of Medical and Sanitary Services for 1948,

> [T]he institution of medical care is a responsibility of the Central Government. A national medical service offers free outdoor medical treatment to the people. With regard to indoor treatment it is free to the poorer classes but a small charge is made in the case of certain income groups. A charge of 30 cents per diem is made from those patients with incomes between Rs.50 and Rs.83 per mensem for accommodation in a non-paying ward. Where the income exceeds Rs.83 per mensem a charge of 50 cents is made. (Wickramasinghe 1949, p. C7)

Rannan-Eliya and de Mel (1997), using data from the 1953 Consumer Finance Survey, found that 90 percent of the population was at a consumption level of less than Rs.600 per year. On this basis, they argued that in the 1940s, when this fee structure was in existence, more than 97 percent of the rural population would have been exempt.

The information from the *Administration Report* was complemented by interviews with key informants, which were carried out with past and present staff of the MOH, including providers, managers, and policymakers up to the ministerial level. The key informants uniformly reported that user fees would in no instance have served as a barrier to access to care: clients unable to pay for services would have received care in the general, "non-paying" wards, which offered a similar level of care but a lower level of comfort than the paying wards.

The absence of user fees was corroborated by an analysis of the health service revenue data reported in *Administration Reports* for several years during the 1950s. In this analysis it was found that revenue collected represented less than the equivalent of 1 percent of total expenditures, implying that the policy of charging clients was applied only occasionally.

Fees for Drugs and Supplies and Other Informal Payments. The government policy of universal free access to health care included all costs, including drugs and supplies. The key informants indicated that since at least the 1950s, this policy has been implemented as intended at all levels of the system: clients would never be charged for drugs or supplies, nor would they be expected to make any other payment. The veracity of this claim was supported by the key informants' repeated reports of the high levels of motivation and job satisfaction experienced by the PHM teams, despite their low wages and extremely difficult working conditions.

Paying for Emergency Referral within the Health System. Ambulances and other vehicles linked to hospitals were called upon to handle emergency referral from maternity homes or primary Health Units to referral hospitals. According to the key informants, in situations in which no ambulance or other vehicle was available, health personnel were normally able to locate and pay for alternate means of transportation, such as taxis or private vehicles, for which the MOH would pay.

Conclusion

Sri Lanka has achieved a remarkably high maternal health status despite its weak economic status. The purpose of this study was to derive lessons from the past for other developing countries that are at earlier phases of health systems development. Several issues in Sri

Lanka today point to the need for health sector reform. Despite those issues, maternal mortality has continued to decline during the past several decades. The challenge today is to ensure that future development does not undermine past achievements.

Notes

1. "Ceylonese" is the previous nomenclature for Sri Lankans.

2. Payroll costs include salaries, cost-of-living allowances, contributions to retirement funds, holiday pay, and railway warrants (vouchers or written authorization for use of railway services).

3. Nonpayroll costs include client diets, drugs, dressings, disinfectants, instruments, equipment, travel costs, laundry, electricity, rent, stationery, office furniture, office requisites, honoraria to blood transfusion donors, propaganda (that is, propagation of information and practices), information, incidental expenses, maintenance costs, uniforms, training expenses, and scholarships.

4. Unrelated expenditures include prevention of malaria and other infectious diseases, grants and rebates payable under the Medical Wants Ordinance, and occupational therapy.

5. Government institutions include small maternity homes and cottage hospitals where deliveries are managed by PHMs and nurse-midwives, secondary-level institutions are hospitals where doctors are available to provide nonsurgical interventions when complications arise, and tertiary-level institutions have obstetricians and surgeons capable of providing comprehensive obstetric care. In all institutions, midwives and nurses manage most uncomplicated births.

6. "Sisters" are nurses who have additional qualifications and training.

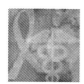

APPENDIX 1

Data Availability and Quality in Malaysia

Maternal Mortality Data

During the 1950s and 1960s, causes of maternal death were recorded only for those deaths that occurred after the woman went to the hospital. At that time, only about 30 percent of births had skilled attendance, and the cause of death was known for about one in every two reported maternal deaths. Even in 1998 only 44 percent of all deaths were medically certified. Maternal deaths accounted for about 10 percent of reported deaths in women in the reproductive age group during 1957–70. The reported maternal death rate continued to fall to about 6 percent in the 1970s, and it reached 2 percent by 1991. During the 1970s, government midwives working in rural areas instituted a practice of visiting those families that had reported a female death to the local Registrar General (RG), to assess whether it was a maternal death, and to determine the factors that contributed to the death. During the next two decades, the system was expanded and strengthened, and by the early 1980s the Ministry of Health (MOH) was aware of more deaths associated with pregnancy and childbirth than the RG's count. However, the RG continued to be the official source of data on maternal deaths, and all official records use the RG data. It was only in the early 1990s that the RG's system was revised to take into account the deaths known to the

153

MOH, and this could partially explain the recorded slowing of the maternal mortality rate decline in the 1990s.

Health Services and Utilization Data

Prior to Independence in 1957, each of the component states in Malaysia had its own health management system, and health system information was not standardized or collated to cover the thirteen states that eventually became Malaysia. Urban local authorities provided most community-based services related to maternal health and kept their own records. State governments maintained hospital data; private sector data was not collected. Although information systems improved during 1957–79, there are some major data gaps in health services and their utilization during the 1970s, and information from urban local authorities and the private sector was not standardized with that of the MOH. After 1980, the federal MOH standardized the monitoring system nationwide, including the public and private sectors, and information generated by the system compares very well with data obtained through nationwide household sample surveys. (It should be noted that this study does not include the two states on the island of Borneo—Sarawak and Sabah—which joined Malaysia at a later stage, and had information systems that lagged.)

Health Expenditure Data and Affordability

Materials

The estimation process used published sources; therefore, there is no question of confidentiality regarding the data and information used. Information was gleaned from many sources: including the published five-year plans of Malaya and Malaysia; *Annual Reports* of the Ministry of Health Malaysia and its predecessor the Medical Department of the Federation of Malay; *Annual Reports* of the Auditor General; annual reports of relevant municipalities; annual reports of university hospital services; *Indicators for Monitoring and*

Evaluation of Strategy of Health for All by the Year 2000 of the Ministry of Health Malaysia; *Malaysia Economic Statistics - Time Series - 1999* of the Department of Statistics Malaysia; *Vital Statistics* of the Department of Statistics Malaysia; schemes of service of the Federation of Malaya; other schedules of salaries of the government employees of Malaysia; *Annual Reports* of the Federation of Malaya; *Official Year Books* of Malaysia of the Government of Malaysia; *Year Books of Statistics* of the Department of Statistics, Malaysia; and several World Bank reports.

Expression of Expenditures in Proportion of GDP

A study of this nature that deals with long periods of time and aims to provide a measure of the affordability of the expenditures involved must deal with two issues: price inflation and the different purchasing power of currencies in relation to their domestic market. The use of GDP as the standard has the merit of relating expenditures to the total resources available in the country at that point in time, and therefore provides a good measure of resource allocation. Using GDP as the standard also overcomes the problem of inflationary forces over time. In addition, unlike foreign exchange rates, which reflect the relative value of the national currency in foreign trade, GDP is concerned with domestic resources and allows for comparisons in efforts of different countries in terms of their available resources. Another device for international comparison would be the use of purchasing power parities; however, these data are available for only some of the years covered by this study.

Estimation of Capital Expenditures

The estimation process took 5-year estimates of actual capital expenditures for public health services contained in the various five-year plans for Malaya and Malaysia. The figures provided aggregates for the whole public health sector and also for specific programs such as rural health services, hospitals, and training. Apportionment based on relative weights was made for training and hospital services. For earlier periods, estimates of aggregates for capital expenditures for the whole public health sector in the annual reports of the Medical Department were used, as they included more complete data on capital expenditures by both central and state governments.

Operating Expenditures

The estimation process of operating expenditures focused on three major components: (a) health services provided by the MOH Malaysia, (b) services supplied by municipalities, and (c) hospital services rendered by the Ministry of Education. There were two major parts to the estimation process: the first was concerned with the aggregate operating expenditure of the public sector as a whole, and the second with the estimation of operating expenditures related to skilled attendance. In turn, the latter had two elements, (1) MCH services by MOH and municipalities and (2) hospital services for skilled attendance in MOH and university hospitals.

In order to provide a clearer picture of trends, five-year aggregates were used that were built up from yearly information. In the estimation of the public health sector expenditure as a whole, interpolation was used in some instances where there was missing data for given years. In other cases, data for representative years in given 5-year periods were used. However, no useful data was available from MOH for the 5-year period of 1966–70, and this led to a gap in the time-series.

The estimation of expenditures for MCH services for the municipalities used data in annual reports related to maternal and child welfare units. Interpolation was used to fill in the information gaps. In the estimation of MCH operating expenditures by MOH, reports on actual expenditures by program and activities were used. There was no information regarding the specific staff employed by the different programs and activities; therefore, it was not possible to follow an estimation path that would use staff as a major component. The reported expenditure was specific for MCH and other activities. Apportionment to MCH was made for training (there were specific figures for this), pharmacy, research and planning, as well as for District Health and central administration.

As in the case of MCH, an apportionment was added to MOH acute hospital expenditures for ancillary functions provided by central units and administration. The estimation of MOH hospital expenditures for skilled attendance at deliveries and the complications of pregnancy relied on aggregated data from acute care hospitals and their admissions for normal and complicated deliveries, and complications of pregnancy. An assumption was made that a normal delivery would involve 1.5 days stay and that a complication would reflect what the hospital allocated for that given period. A study carried out in Malaysia concerned with average lengths of stay for different causes of admission to public hospitals shows that the lengths of stay used in this estimation are substantially higher than those in that study. Therefore, the estimates made are an upper limit of the actual situation. The aggregate of the patient days for these two admission scenarios was used to estimate the proportion of patient days related to skilled assistance of the total number of patient days in MOH acute hospitals. This proportion was then applied to the aggregate total MOH acute hospital expenditure, to arrive at the expenditure attributable to normal and complicated deliveries, and complications of pregnancy. The estimation related to university hospital services used figures from annual reports that included average length of stay for obstetric patients and the number admitted for this service. An additional estimate was made for some complications of pregnancy not admitted to obstetric wards. Again, the proportion of the number of days involved for these admissions was used to estimate the expenditure related to normal and complicated deliveries, and complications of pregnancy.

In the estimation of skilled attendance services for MOH, there were no useful figures available for the years prior to the 1970s. Data for the years 1973–75 and 1976–77 were used to represent the relevant five-year periods. There was another gap to 1985; Auditor General reports provided specific information for the years from 1985–95. The data for 1985 was used to represent the five-year period 1980–85, and aggregates for the following years were used for the following two five-year periods. The estimated expenditures were then related to GDP at current prices for the relevant years, so that expenditures in terms of their proportion of GDP could be estimated. The same system was used to estimate university hospital services and MCH supplied by the municipalities.

Data Availability and Quality in Sri Lanka

Maternal Mortality Data Availability and Quality

Intensive review of data sources used in previous studies showed that some of the previously quoted data required correction. The data used in this study are from the reports published by the Registrar General (RG). Birth and death registration has been studied for 1953, 1967, and in 1980 and has been found to be 89 percent, 95 percent, and 93 percent complete, respectively (Sri Lanka, Ministry of Health, 1993). However, in recent years, the quality of data has deteriorated because of the civil war in the north and east; studies have revealed a degree of underregistration of deaths.

A study carried out in 1994–95 showed that maternal deaths in the Western Province were 24 percent underreported (Bandhutila-ka, 1996). It has been suggested that the discrepancy between the maternal death reviews and those officially registered has increased in recent years (De Silva, 2001). The increasing discrepancy may be a result of more indirect causes of maternal death being reported in recently through the field and hospital systems, following the refresher education of health personnel on the definition of maternal mortality and the importance of reporting it.

Health Service Data Quality

Health service data for the period 1900–57 are available from the reports of the Director of Health Services, and since 1980, from the *Annual Health Bulletin*. There are gaps in health service data during the period 1968–79, when health data were included in the general administrative reports, which did not give adequate details for the present study. Unpublished data available from the Medical Statistics Unit have been used to supplement the above sources. Health service data do not include any information from the private sector. The births reported are only those occurring in government institutions; this too may be incomplete because data from the northeastern province are not available.

The numbers of registered doctors, nurses, and midwives are available from the Sri Lanka Medical Council for 1907, 1949, and 1930 respectively. Nurses with midwifery qualifications are entered in the register both under nurses and under midwives.

Information was also obtained from 15 key informants. These informants included doctors, nurses, and midwives who had worked in health services at the district level and had become senior managers subsequently; one had become a minister of health. The interviews covered issues such as perceptions regarding maternal and child health services and obstetric practices in the late 1950s to the 1970s, the acceptance of midwives, the back-up services they had, and training during the early periods.

Expenditure and Affordability

The data used to estimate the expenditure on skilled attendance are mainly from the *Annual Reports* of the director general of Health Services, complemented by data from other published reports. For the period 1932–54, the annual *Administration Reports* issued by the Director General of Health Services provided comprehensive data on expenditure and admissions. For 1955–62, the reports issued by the Director General of Health Services provided aggregate recurrent expenditure figures. The decades of the 1960s and 1970s proved to be the most difficult in terms of expenditure data, since detailed annual administration reports were not issued; for this period health expenditure data was calculated using the ratio health expenditure-to-GDP (1963–72) and government health expenditure-to-GDP (1973–79) as published by the Central Bank. During the period 1980–99, the *Annual Health Bulletin* proved to be a most valuable source of health expenditure and admissions data.

For each year under study, total expenditure was calculated on the basis of payroll data[1] and other expenditure data[2] available in the annual reports. Whenever possible, expenditures unrelated to maternal care[3] were excluded. Despite attempts to disaggregate payroll cost by staffing category (e.g., midwives, public health midwives, etc.), the lack of detailed data in all but the most recent years dictated that the expenditure on skilled attendance would be calculated by allocating total expenditure to maternity and non-maternity functions by the ratio of maternity to nonmaternity admissions.

In assessing the affordability to clients and households, information on policy was found in the annual administration reports and other published sources, which was complemented by information gathered in key informant interviews carried out in Colombo in June 2001.

Notes

1. Payroll cost includes personal emoluments, cost of living allowances, "provident fund" contributions, holiday pay, and railway warrants.

2. Non-payroll cost includes client diets, drugs, dressings, disinfectants, instruments, equipment, travelling and transport cost, laundry, electricity, rent, stationery, office furniture, office requisites, honoraria to blood transfusion donors, propaganda, information, incidental expenses, maintenance cost, uniforms, and training expenses and scholarships.

3.   Prevention of malaria and other infectious diseases, grants and rebates payable under the Medical Wants Ordinance, Occupational therapy.

Assessment of Affordability

Methodological Approach

Estimation of Expenditures versus Costing

This study has used the estimation of expenditures rather than the estimation of costs. There are both conceptual and practical reasons for this decision: first, countries that need to embark on similar efforts should have the financial resources to undertake the task; for instance, a costing approach would have apportioned capital costs over the future life of assets acquired. However, countries will need to make the disbursement up front. Therefore, the costing approach would underestimate the dimensions of the initial financial resources required, especially in an expanding system, and then overestimate capital outlays as the system matures. It is important to consider that it is not possible to go back in time and conduct a costing study of the services involved in the 1970s and 1980s because of the lack of relevant information.

Estimation and Uncertainty

This study has taken the approach that if there was to be a misstatement of the value of the estimates, it would be preferable to be on the high side rather than on the low side. Therefore, the estimates produced have attempted to include significant expenditures incurred throughout the MOH to ensure that the services were provided. When there was some uncertainty regarding the basis of estimation, an attempt was made to take the high side. Consequently, the estimates could be considered as an upper limit of the expenditures actually incurred.

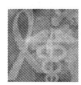

APPENDIX 4

Key Informants

Key Informants in Malaysia

NAME	KEY PROFESSIONAL POSITIONS	PERIOD	INSTITUTION(S)
Abu Bakar Suleiman	• Medical officer at district and general hospitals • Consultant physician • Director general, Health	1975–2001	Ministry of Health
Abdul Khalid Sahan	• Medical officer of health at district level • Director of health services at state level • Director of several national level programs • Director general, Health	1961–1989	Ministry of Health
Raja Ahmad Nordin	• Medical officer of health at district level • Director, Public Health Institute • Director, Health Services • Director general, Health	1950s–1980s	Ministry of Health
Raj Karim	• Medical officer • Director, Maternal and Child Health (national level)	1971–2000	Ministry of Health
M. S. Murthy	• Nurse tutor • Senior nursing manager (national level)	1956–1983	Ministry of Health
Rebecca John	• Nurse–midwife at health centers • Nursing trainer • Successive promotional positions at state, hospital, and national levels	1968–1994	Ministry of Health
Ajima Hassan	• Nurse–midwife at health centers • Various promotional positions at district, state, and national levels	1968–2000	Ministry of Health
S. Maheswaran	• Consultant obstetrician in hospitals in several states	1960s–2000	Ministry of Health
T. Ng Khoon Fong	• Consultant obstetrician in hospitals in several states	1961–1978	Ministry of Health
Alex Mathews	• Consultant obstetrician in hospitals in several states	1970s–2001	Ministry of Health
Jegasothy Ravindran	• Consultant obstetrician in hospitals in several states	1980s to date	Ministry of Health

166

A.Tharmaratnam	• Consultant obstetrician in hospitals in several states	1958–1974	Ministry of Health
Ali Hamzah	• Administrative officer, Social Sector	1980s–1990s	Economic Planning Unit, Prime Minister's Department
K. Kananatu	• Administrative officer, Social Sector	1970s–1990s	Economic Planning Unit, Prime Minister's Department

Key Informants in Sri Lanka

NAME	KEY PROFESSIONAL POSITIONS	PERIOD	INSTITUTION(S)
Akkarakkuruppu Mudiyanselage Lokubandara Beligaswatte	• Director general of health	1998–2002	• Ministry of Health
Siva Obeyesekere	• Deputy minister of health • Minister of health	1970–1977	Ministry of Health
Godfrey Gunathilleke	• Ceylon Civil Service • Ministry of Planning and Economic Affairs • WHO Taskforce on Health and Development • Founder member and head of Marga Institute • Has researched and published extensively on health and socioeconomic development in Sri Lanka	1950–1998	• Ministry of Local Government • Ministry of Planning • WHO • Marga Institute, Sri Lanka (an independent research organization)
Joe Fernando	• District medical officer • Medical officer of health • Medical superintendent, provincial hospital • Superintendent, Health Services in two provinces (equivalent to current provincial director of Health) • Deputy director general, Public Health Services • Director general, Health Services • Secretary, Health	1956–1994	Ministry of Health

(continued on next page)

Key Informants in Sri Lanka (Continued)

NAME	KEY PROFESSIONAL POSITIONS	PERIOD	INSTITUTION(S)
Nimal W. Vidyasagara	• Medical officer • Assistant medical officer of health • Medical officer, Maternal and Child Health • Medical officer, Family Health Bureau • Director, Maternal and Child Health • Head, Family Health Bureau • Regional advisor, Maternal and Child Health SEARO • National programme coordinator, WHO office, Colombo	1961–1995	Ministry of Health WHO, Southeast Asia Regional Office
Hiranthi Wijemanne	• Programme officer; worked in the field of maternal and child health	1970–2001	UNICEF
Kusum Wickramasuriya	• Medical officer, Health • Medical officer, Maternal and Child Health • Medical officer, Family Health Bureau • Director, Maternal and Child Health	1967–1998	Ministry of Health
Sybil Wijesinghe	• Medical officer, Health • Medical officer, Maternal and Child Health • Medical officer, Family Health Bureau • UNICEF consultant, Family Health Bureau	1968–2002	Ministry of Health
Gamalath	• Nurse • Public health nursing sister • Public health nursing tutor, Family Health Bureau	1950–1992	Ministry of Health
Team from the National Institute of Health Science[a]: Dulcie de Silva H.M.S.K. Amunugama	• Director • Deputy director, Training, Public Health Midwives, Public Health Nursing Sisters and Tutors	1970s–2002	Ministry of Health

168

Name	Positions	Years	Organization
N. C. de Costa	• Staff nurse • Sister tutor • Senior tutor • Principal, School of Nursing • Director, Nursing Education	1960–1999	Ministry of Health
Lakshman Senanayaka	• Medical officer, peripheral and district hospitals • Senior house officer, Obstetrics and Gynaecology • Registrar, Obstetrics and Gynaecology • Consultant obstetrician and gynecologist at base hospitals and provincial hospitals • Consultant obstetrician and gynecologist at teaching hospitals	1969–2002	Ministry of Health
Anoma Jayathilake	• Medical officer, district hospital • Medical officer of health • Medical officer, Maternal and Child Health • Medical officer, National Institute of Health Science • Medical officer, Family Health Bureau • Specialist medical officer, Family Health Bureau • In charge of maternal mortality review and data	1984–to date	Ministry of Health
Nandrani de Zoysa	• Medical officer • Medical officer, National Blood Bank • Director, National Blood Transfusion Services	1961–1994	Ministry of Health

[a]The National Institute of Health Science is the premier center of the Department of Health Services for training personnel required for the Primary Health Care programme. The institution is located in the first Health Unit (established in 1926) and has taken on and expanded the training functions undertaken by that Health Unit.

References

Abdul, Majid. 1971. *Rural Health*. Kuala Lumpur: Ministry of Health Malaysia.

Abdul, Wahab, Gurmukh Singh, Martinez. 1974. *Regionalisation of Patient Care Services in Malaysia*. Kuala Lumpur: Government Printers.

Abeyesundere, A.N.A. 1976. *Recent Trends in Malaria Morbidity and Mortality in Sri Lanka. Population Problems of Sri Lanka*. Colombo: Demographic Training and Research Unit, University of Colombo.

AbouZahr, C., and T. Wardlaw. 2001. "Maternal Mortality at the End of a Decade: Signs of Progress?" *Bulletin of the World Health Organization* 79: 32–34.

Abu Bakar, S., A. Mathews, R. Jegasothy, R. Ali, and N. Kandiah. 1999. "Strategy for Reducing Maternal Mortality." *Bulletin of the World Health Organization* 77(2): 190–93.

Abu Bakar, S., and M. Jegathesan. 2000. *Health in Malaysia. Achievements and Challenges*. Kuala Lumpur: Planning and Development Division, Ministry of Health Malaysia.

Administration Report of the Director of Medical and Sanitary Services 1951. 1952. Colombo: Ceylon Government Press.

Administration Report of the Director of Medical and Sanitary Service 1962. 1963. Colombo: Ceylon Government Press.

Alailima, P. 1997. "Social Policy in SriLanka." In Lakshman (ed.), *Dilemmas of Development: Fifty Years of Economic Change in Sri Lanka*. Colombo: Sri Lanka Association of Economists, pp. 127–70.

Alam, I., and J. Cleland. 1981. "Illustrative Analysis: Recent Fertility Trends in Sri Lanka." In *World Fertility Survey* 15. London: Scientific Reports.

Amarasinghe, P.H. 1962. "Measures to Reduce Maternal Mortality in Ceylon." *Ceylon Medical Journal* 7(3–4): 153–174.

Association of Obstetricians and Gynaecologists of Ceylon. 1969. "Recommendations for the Reduction of Maternal Mortality in Ceylon: Memorandum on the Reduction of Maternal Deaths in Ceylon Submitted by the Association of Obstetricians and Gynaecologists of Ceylon to the Hon'able Minister of Health." *Journal of the Association of Obstetricians and Gynaecologists of Ceylon*: 45–49.

Auditor General. 1985–1995. *Akaun Awam Lengkap Malaysia*. Kuala Lumpur.

Bandhutilaka, T.H.C. 1996. "Epidemiology of Maternal Mortality in Sri Lanka." M.D. thesis. Colombo: Post Graduate Institute of Medicine, University of Colombo.

Bindusara, T.H.C. 2000. "Voluntary Blood Donation—Country Scenario in Sri Lanka." Proceedings of the International Conference on Safe Blood Transfusion Practices. Colombo: Ministry of Health.

Borghi, J. 2000. "A Case Study of the Relationship between Health Sector Development and Reproductive Health: Sri Lanka." Unpublished paper prepared for the World Bank, Washington, D.C.

Caldwell, J., K.H.W. Gaminirathne, P. Caldwell, S. De Silva, B. Caldwell, N. Weeraratne, and P. Silva. 1987. "The Role of Traditional Fertility Regulations in Sri Lanka." *Studies in Family Planning* 18: 1–20.

Campbell, O. 2001. "What Are Maternal Health Policies in Developing Countries and Who Drives Them? A Review of the Last Half-Century." *Studies in Health Services Organisation and Policy* 17: 415–48.

Central Bank of Ceylon. 1968–1984. *Annual Reports*. Colombo.

Central Bank of Sri Lanka. 1986–1999. *Annual Reports*. Colombo.

Chellappah, S.F. 1949. *Administration Report of the Director of Medical and Sanitary Services for 1948*. Colombo: Ceylon Government Press.

Chong, Ah Foo. 1971. *The Development of Nursing Programmes in West Malaysia 1963–1970*. Nursing Division, Ministry of Health Malaysia.

City Council of George Town. 1946–1960, 1984. *Annual Reports of the City Council of George Town*. Penang.

———. 1963, 1974. *Budget*. Penang.

Claeson, M., C.C. Griffin, T.A. Johnston, M. McLachlan, A.B. Soucat, A. Wagstaff, and A.S. Yazbeck. 2001. *Poverty Reduction and the Health Sector.* Washington, D.C.: World Bank.

Daga, A.S., and S.R. Daga. 1993. "Epidemiology of Perinatal Loss in Rural Maharashtra." *Journal of Tropical Paediatrics* 39 (April): 83–85.

De Brouwere, V., R. Tonglet, and W. Van Lerberghe. 1998. "Strategies for Reducing Maternal Mortality in Developing Countries: What Can We Learn from the History of the Industrialized West?" *Tropical Medicine and International Health* 3(10): 771–82.

De Brouwere, V., and W. Van Lerberghe (eds.). 2001. "Safe Motherhood Strategies: A Review of Evidence." *Studies in Health Services Organisation and Policy* 17: 1–448.

De Silva, A., K.C.S. Dalpatadu, S.M. Samarage, and A.M. Das. 1997. *Assessment of the Prospects of Paying Wards in Government Hospitals as Complementary Financing for Hospitals.* Colombo: World Health Organization.

De Silva, D.M. 1956. *Health Progress in Ceylon.* Colombo: Ministry of Health.

De Silva, S. 2001. "Maternal Mortality in Sri Lanka: Estimation, Levels, Trends and Causes." *Sri Lanka Journal of Population Studies* 4: 49–63.

Dissanayake, L. 1999. "Factors Influencing Stabilisation of Women's Age at Marriage in Sri Lanka." *Demography of Sri Lanka: Issues and Challenges.* Colombo: Department of Demography, University of Colombo.

Donnay, F. 2000. "Maternal Survival in Developing Countries: What Can be Done in the Next Decade." *International Journal of Gynecology and Obstetrics* 70: 89–97.

Fadil, A. 1997. *Poverty Reduction in Malaysia, 1970–1995: Major Features.* Paper presented to the Regional Steering Committee on the Economic Advancement of Rural and Island Women in Asia Pacific Region.

Federation of Malaya. Various years. *Annual Reports of the Medical Department.* Kuala Lumpur: Government Press.

———. 1951, 1952, 1955. *Annual Report.* Kuala Lumpur.

———. 1961, 1964, 1967, 1970, 1975. *Official Year Book.* Kuala Lumpur: Government Printers.

Fernando, L. 1996. "Development of Maternity Services in Sri Lanka." *Sri Lanka Journal of Obstetrics and Gynaecology* 18: 3–8.

Fernando, M.A. 1994. *Sex Differentials in Mortality in Sri Lanka*. Peradeniya: University of Peradeniya.

Frankenberg, E., and D. Thomas. 2001. "Women's Health and Pregnancy Outcomes: Do Services Make a Difference?" *Demography* 38(2): 53–65.

Fullerton, J., and A. Thompson (eds.). Forthcoming. *Skilled during Childbirth. A Review of the Evidence*. New York: Family Care International.

Goodburn, E., and O. Campbell. 2001. "Reducing Maternal Mortality in the Developing Countries: Sector-Wide Approaches May be the Key." *British Medical Journal* 322(April): 917–20.

Government of Malaysia. 1936, 1939. *Malayan Year Book*. Singapore: Government Printers.

———. 1991. *Second Outline Perspective Plan 1991–2000*. Kuala Lumpur: National Printing Department.

———. 2000. *Third Outline Perspective Plan 2000–2010*. Kuala Lumpur: National Printing Press.

———. Various years. *Five Year Malaysia Plan (1966–1970, 1971–1975, 1976–1980, 1981–1985, 1986–1990, 1991–1995, 1996–2000, 2001–2005)*. Kuala Lumpur: Government Printers.

Graham, W.J., J.S. Bell, and C.H. Bullough. 2001. "Can Skilled Attendance at Delivery Reduce Maternal Mortality in Developing Countries?" *Studies in Health Organisation and Policy* 17: 97–130.

Gunatilleke, G. 1984. "Intersectoral Linkages in Health Development." Geneva: World Health Organization. Processed.

———. 2000. "Sri Lanka's Social Achievements and Challenges in Social Development and Public Policy." In Dharam Ghar (ed.), *Social Development and Public Policy: A Study of Some Successful Experiences*. London: U.N. Research Institute for Social Development. Handmills and London: Macmillan Press Ltd.

Gunesekara, S.T. 1938. *Administration Report of the Director of Medical and Sanitary Services 1937*. Colombo: Ceylon Government Press.

Hammer, J.S., I. Nabi, and J.A. Cerone. 1995. "Distributional Effects of Social Sector Expenditures in Malaysia, 1974–89." In D. van de Walle and K. Nead (eds.), *Public Spending and the Poor*. Baltimore: The Johns Hopkins University Press.

Herath-Guneratne, V.T. 1965. *Administration Report of the Director of Medical and Sanitary Services 1962–63*. Colombo: Ceylon Government Press.

Hill, K., C. AbouZahr, and T. Wardlaw. 2001. "Estimates of Maternal Mortality for 1995." *Bulletin of the World Health Organization* 79(3): 182–93.

Hogberg, U., and S. Wall. 1986. "Secular Trends in Maternal Mortality in Sweden from 1750 to 1980." *Bulletin of the World Health Organization* 64(1): 79–84.

Hoj, L., J. Stensballe, and P. Aaby. 1999. "Maternal Mortality in Guinea-Bissau—the Use of Verbal Autopsy in a Multi-Ethnic Population." *International Journal of Epidemiology* 28(1): 70–76.

Hospital Universiti. 1981–95. *Annual Reports*. Kuala Lumpur: University of Malaya.

Hsiao, W. 2000. *A Preliminary Assessment of Sri Lanka's Health Sector and Steps Forward*. Cambridge, Mass.: Harvard University and Institute of Policy Studies.

IBRD (International Bank for Reconstruction and Development). 1952. "Economic Development of Ceylon." Part 2 of Selected Fields of Development: Report of a mission organized by IBRD at the request of the Government of Ceylon. Colombo: Ceylon Government Press.

———. 1955. *The Economic Development of Malaya*. Baltimore: The Johns Hopkins University Press.

Jayawardene, C.H.S., and S. Selvaratnam. 1967. "Fertility Level and Trends in Ceylon." Contributed paper. Sydney: International Union for Scientific Study of Population Conference.

Jones, G.W., and S. Selvaratnam. 1972. *Population Growth and Economic Development in Ceylon*. Colombo: Hansa Publishers in association with Marga Institute.

Jowett, M. 2000. "Cost-Effective Safe Motherhood Interventions in Low-Income Countries: a Review." Discussion Paper 181. Centre for Health Economics: The University of York.

Kaunitz, A.M., C. Spence, T.S. Danielson, R.W. Rochat, and D.A. Grimes. 1984. "Perinatal and Maternal Mortality in a Religious Group Avoiding Obstetric Care." *American Journal of Obstetrics and Gynecology* 150(7): 26–31.

Kennedy, J. 1993. *A History of Malaysia*, 3rd ed. Kuala Lumpur: Abdul Majeed & Co.

Koblinski, M.A., O. Campbell, and J. Heichelheim. 1999. "Organizing Delivery Care: What Works for Safe Motherhood?" *Bulletin of the World Health Organization* 77(5): 399–406.

Kuala Lumpur City Council. 1954, 1960–1985. *Annual Reports of the Municipality of Kuala Lumpur*.

————. 1985–1995. *Annual Reports, Department of Health.*

Kuala Lumpur City Hall. 1991–1993. *Budget.*

Liljestrand, J. 2000. "Strategies to Reduce Maternal Mortality Worldwide." Current opinion in *Obstetrics and Gynecology* 12(6): 513–17.

Malaya. 1955. "The Midwives Ordinance 1954." In *Federal Ordinances and State and Settlements Enactments Passed During the Year 1954.* Kuala Lumpur: Government Printers.

Malayan Union. 1946–1960. *Reports of the Medical Department for the Year.* Kuala Lumpur: Government Printers.

Malaysia. 1968. "The Midwives Act 1966." In *Acts of Parliament Passed During the Year 1966.* Kuala Lumpur: Government Printers.

————. 1971. "The Midwives (Registration) Regulations 1971." In *His Majesty's Government Gazette* 15. Kuala Lumpur: Government Printers.

————. 1972. *Laws of Malaysia, Act A 109, Midwives Amendment Act.* Kuala Lumpur: Government Printers.

————. 1985. "Nurses Act 1950. Nurses Regulations 1985." In *His Majesty's Government Gazette* 22. Kuala Lumpur: Government Printers.

————. 1990. "The Midwives Act 1966. Midwives Regulations 1990." In *His Majesty's Government Gazette* 15. Kuala Lumpur: Government Printers.

Malaysia, Department of Statistics. 1970. *Annual Statistics Bulletin: Peninsular Malaysia 1970.* Kuala Lumpur: Government Printers.

————. Various years. *Social Statistics Bulletin.* Kuala Lumpur: Government Printers.

————. Various years. *Vital Statistics Report.* Kuala Lumpur.

————. 1991. *Vital Statistics Time Series: Peninsular Malaysia 1911–1985.* Kuala Lumpur: Government Printers.

————. 1999. *Malaysia Economic Statistics—Time Series—1999.* Kuala Lumpur.

————. 2001. *Compilations 1966–2001.* Kuala Lumpur.

————. 2001. *Maternal Mortality by States in Malaysia 1955–1999.* Kuala Lumpur (Compilation by Department of Statistics).

Malaysia, Ministry of Health. 1987–1997. *Indicators for Monitoring and Evaluation of Strategy for Health for All by the Year 2000*. Kuala Lumpur: Health Information and Documentation Unit.

———. 1991. "Report of National Meeting on Maternal Mortality." Kuala Lumpur.

———. 1992. "Report on National Review Meeting, Maternal and Child Health Programme." Genting Highlands.

———. 1994, 1997. "Report on the Confidential Enquiries into Maternal Deaths in Malaysia for the Year 1992." Kuala Lumpur.

———. 1998. "Evaluation of Implementation of the Confidential Enquiries into Maternal Deaths in the Improvement of Maternal Health Services." Kuala Lumpur.

———. Various years. *Annual Report of Ministry of Health Malaysia*. Kuala Lumpur.

——— and UNICEF. 1994. *Report of National Maternal Mortality Conference*. Port Dickson.

Malaysia. Ministry of National Unity and Social Development. 1999. *Population Profile Malaysia*. Kuala Lumpur: National Population and Family Development Board.

Malaysia. National Population and Family Development Board. 1986. *District Level Differences in Maternal Mortality Rates, Peninsular Malaysia*. Population Research Series No. 2.

Manderson, L. 1996. *Sickness and the State, Health and Illness in Colonial Malaya, 1870–1940*. Cambridge, UK: Cambridge University Press.

Marga Institute. 1984. *Intersectoral Action for Health: Sri Lanka Study*. Colombo.

Mbaruku, G., and S. Bergstrom. 1995. "Reducing Maternal Mortality in Kigoma, Tanzania." *Health Policy and Planning* 10(1): 71–8.

Meegama, S.A. 1969. "Decline in Maternal and Infant Mortality in Relation to Malaria Eradication." *Population Studies* 23(2): 289–302.

Ministry of Health Sri Lanka. 1997. *Annual Health Bulletin 1996*. Colombo.

Myrdal, G. 1968. *Asian Drama, Vol. 1*. New York: Pantheon Books.

Nadarajah, T. 1976. "Trends and Differentials in Mortality." In *Population of Sri Lanka, 1976.* Country Monograph Series No. 4. Bangkok: Economic and Social Commission for Asia and the Pacific.

Nahar, S., and A. Costello. 1998. "The Hidden Cost of 'Free' Maternity Care in Dhaka, Bangladesh." *Health Policy and Planning* 13(4): 417–22.

Newman, P. 1965. *Malaria Eradication and Population Growth.* Ann Arbor, Michigan: School of Public Health.

Noordin, Raja A. 1978. "Primary Health Care in the Underserved Areas with Special Reference to Malaysia." Proceedings of Intercountry Workshop on Primary Health Care in Malaysia and Republic of Korea. Kuala Lumpur: Ministry of Health Malaysia and WHO, November 13–18.

Nor, Laily Aziz, Tan Boon Ann, and Kuan Liu Chee. 1977. *The Malaysian National Family Planning Programme: Some Facts and Figures.* Kuala Lumpur: National Family Planning Board Malaysia.

Nursing Division. 1988. "Historical Perspective in Nursing Service and Nursing Education in Malaysia." Kuala Lumpur: Ministry of Health. Processed.

Pathmanathan, I., (ed.). 1977. *Report of Maternal Health and Early Pregnancy Wastage.* Kuala Lumpur: Federation of Family Planning Associations.

Pathmanathan, I., and S. Dhairiam. 1990. "Malaysia: Moving from Infectious to Chronic Diseases." In E. Tarimo and A. Creese (eds.), *Achieving Health for All by the Year 2000. Midway Reports of Country Experiences.* Geneva: World Health Organization.

Peebles, P. 1982. *Sri Lanka: Handbook of Historical Statistics.* Boston: G.K. Hall & Co.

Perera, N., D. Lellupitiya, and S. Priyanthie. 1999. "A Demographic Profile of Sri Lanka." In *Demography of Sri Lanka: Issues and Challenges.* Colombo: Department of Demography, University of Colombo.

Phua, Kai Hong. 1987. "The Development of Health Services in Malaysia and Singapore 1867–1960." Thesis presented to the London School of Economics and Political Science, University of London.

Public Health Institute. 1983a. *Study of Hospital Utilization in Peninsular Malaysia.* Kuala Lumpur: Ministry of Health Malaysia.

———. 1983b. *Annual Report 1982* and *Development and Achievements from 1966–1981.* Kuala Lumpur: Ministry of Health Malaysia.

———. 1985. *Evaluation of Training for Family Health Services in Peninsular Malaysia.* Kuala Lumpur: Ministry of Health Malaysia.

———. 1987. *Project Completion Report UNFPA Grant MAL/79/PO5. Strengthening of Staff Development and Training for Family Health, Family Planning, Health Education.* Kuala Lumpur: Ministry of Health Malaysia.

———. 1988. *National Health and Morbidity Survey, 1986–1987.* Kuala Lumpur: Ministry of Health Malaysia.

———. 1997. *Report of the Second National Health and Morbidity Survey Conference.* Kuala Lumpur: Ministry of Health Malaysia.

Rahmah, Kassim. 1998. "Malaysia: Continuing Rural Development into the Next Millennium." Paper presented at a workshop on Appropriate Strategies for Poverty Alleviation and Sustainable Development, Institute for Rural Advancement, Ministry of Rural Development, Malaysia, December 7–19.

Raj Karim. 2000. "Malaysia's Experience." Paper presented at the RETA Strengthening Safe Motherhood Programs Projects, Kuala Lumpur.

Raj Karim, J. Ravindran, and Y. Mahani. 2000. "Low Maternal Mortality Country Report on Malaysia." Paper presented at the International Conference on Safe Motherhood, Tunisia, November 13–15.

Ravindran J. and A. Matthews. 1996. "Maternal Mortality in Malaysia 1991–1992: The Paradox of Increased Rates." *Journal of Obstetrics and Gynecology* 16(2): 86–88.

Rannan-Eliya, R.P., and N. de Mel. 1997. *Resource Mobilisation for the Health Sector in Sri Lanka.* Boston: Harvard School of Public Health.

Retherford, R.D., and J.R. Rele. 1989. "A Decomposition of Recent Fertility Changes in South Asia." *Population and Development Review* 15(4): 739–747.

Rodrigo J.N. 1987. "The Changing Pattern of Maternal Mortality in Sri Lanka." *Journal of the Sri Lanka College of Obstetricians and Gynaecologists* 13: 11–40.

Rodrigo J.N., L. Fernando, L. Senanayaka, P. Gunasekara, and S. De Silva. n.d. *Maternal Deaths in Sri Lanka: A Review of Estimates and Causes.* Colombo: Sri Lanka College of Obstetricians and Gynaecologists and UNICEF.

Rohana, Ahmadun. 1986. "Pelaksanaan Projek Pendidikan Kesajahteraan Keluarga Melalui Program Pembangunan Keluarga." Paper presented at the workshop on Kebangsaan Pendidikan Kesahteraan Keluarga, Ministry of National and Rural Development. April.

Ronsmans, C. 2001. "What Is the Evidence of the Role of Audits to Improve the Quality of Obstetric Care?" *Studies in Health Services Organisation and Policy* 17: 207–27.

Sanderatne, N. 2000. "Social Development Since Independence: Early Gains and Later Strains." *Economic Growth and Social Transformations: Five Lectures on Sri Lanka.* Colombo: Tamarind Publications.

Sandosham, A. 1965. *Malariology with Special Reference to Malaya.* Kuala Lumpur: University of Malay Press.

Save the Children USA. 2001. *Save the Children: State of the World's Newborn.* Washington, D.C.

Sen, A. 1999. *Development as Freedom.* New York: Anchor Books.

Seneviratne, H.R., and L.C. Rajapaksa. 2000. "Safe Motherhood in Sri Lanka: A 100-year March." *International Journal of Gynecology and Obstetrics* 70(1): 113–24.

Shiffman, J. 2000. "Can Poor Countries Surmount High Maternal Mortality?" *Studies in Family Planning* 31(4): 274–89.

Simeonov, L.A. 1975. *Better Health for Sri Lanka: Report on a Health Manpower Study.* New Delhi: World Health Organization, Regional Office for South East Asia.

Sri Lanka. Department of Census and Statistics. 1961–1964. *Statistical Abstract of Ceylon.* Colombo: Government Press.

———. 1975. *Statistical Abstract of Sri Lanka 1973.* Colombo: Department of Government Printing.

———. 1977–1999. *Statistical Abstract of the Democratic Socialist Republic of Sri Lanka.* Colombo.

———. 1983. *Sri Lanka Contraceptive Prevalence Survey 1982.* Colombo.

———. 1995. *Demographic and Health Survey Sri Lanka 1993.* Colombo: Ministry of Plan Implementation.

———. 1996. *Statistical Pocket Book of the Democratic Socialist Republic of Sri Lanka.* Colombo.

———. 1998. *Population and Housing Estimates from the Demographic and Health Surveys 1993.* Colombo: Ministry of Finance, Planning, Ethnic Affairs and National Integration.

———. 2001. *Demographic and Health Survey Sri Lanka 2000, Preliminary Report.* Colombo: Ministry of Finance and Planning.

———. 1993. *Annual Health Bulletin 1992.* Colombo: Ministry of Health.

———. 1997. *Annual Health Bulletin 1996.* Colombo: Ministry of Health.

Starrs, A. 1998. *The Safe Motherhood Action Agenda: Priorities for the Next Decade.* New York: Family Care International.

Suffian. 1967. *Report of the Royal Commission on the Revision of Salaries and Conditions of Service in the Public Services.* Kuala Lumpur.

Treffers, P.E., A.A. Olukoya, B.J. Ferguson, and J. Liljestrand. 2001. "Care of Adolescent Pregnancy and Childbirth." *International Journal of Obstetrics and Gynaecology* (75)2: 111–21.

UNDP (United Nations Development Programme). 2000. *Human Development Report 2000.* New York.

UNICEF (United Nations Children's Fund). 1996. *The State of the World's Children 1996.* New York.

UNICEF, WHO (World Health Organization), and UNFPA (United Nations Population Fund). 1997. *Guidelines for Monitoring the Availability and Use of Obstetric Services.* New York: UNFPA.

Uragoda, C.G. 1987. *A History of Medicine in Sri Lanka.* Colombo: Sri Lanka Medical Association.

U.S. Centers for Disease Control and Prevention, U.S. Agency for International Development, Ministry of Health Sri Lanka, and CARE. 1978. *Sri Lanka Nutrition Survey 1975-76.* Atlanta.

Vidyasagara, N.W. 1983. *Family Health Impact Survey 1982.* Colombo: Family Health Bureau, Ministry of Health.

———. 2001. "Health Care in the Plantation Sector." *The Journal of the College of Community Physicians of Sri Lanka* (Millennium supplement): 29–41.

WHO. 1999. "Reduction of Maternal Mortality." A UNFPA/UNICEF/WHO/World Bank Joint Statement. Geneva.

Wickramasinghe W.G. 1949. *Administration Report of the Director of Medical and Sanitary Services for 1948.* Colombo: Ceylon Government Press.

————. 1952. *Administration Report of the Director of Medical and Sanitary Services for 1951.* Colombo: Ceylon Government Press.

Wickramasuriya, G.A.W. 1939. "Maternal Mortality and Morbidity in Ceylon." *Journal of the Ceylon Branch of the British Medical Association* 36(2): 79–106.

World Bank. 1978. *World Development Report 1978.* Washington, D.C.

————. 1981. *World Development Report 1981.* New York: Oxford University Press.

————. 1983. *World Development Report 1983.* New York: Oxford University Press.

————. 1997. *World Development Report 1997.* New York: Oxford University Press.

————. 1999. *Safe Motherhood and the World Bank: Lessons from 10 Years of Experience.* Washington, D.C.

————. 2000. *Attacking Poverty. World Development Report 2000/2001.* Washington, D.C.

————. 2001. *World Development Indicators 2001.* Washington, D.C.

Wright, N.H. 1969. "Maternal Mortality in Ceylon: Trend, Causes and Potential Reduction by Family Planning." *Journal of Obstetrics and Gynaecology of the Association of Obstetricians and Gynaecologists of Ceylon* 42–54.

Young, K., W.C.F. Bussink, and P. Hasan. 1980. *Malaysia Growth and Equity in a Multiracial Society.* Baltimore: The Johns Hopkins University Press.

Breinigsville, PA USA
21 March 2010
234569BV00004B/19/A